Plant Spirit Herbalism

PLANT SPIRIT HERBALISM

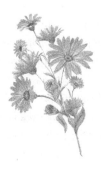

DISCOVER THE POWER OF MEDICINAL HERBS
for Inner Transformation

WENDY DOONER

Hierophantpublishing

This book contains general information about plants that have been traditionally used as herbal remedies. It is not intended to be used as a medical reference. Consult your doctor before using any of the remedies in this book, especially if you are pregnant, breastfeeding, have an existing medical condition, or are taking prescription drugs.

Copyright © 2025 by Wendy Dooner

All rights reserved, including the right to reproduce this work in any form whatsoever, without permission in writing from the publisher, except for brief passages in connection with a review.

Cover design by Sky Peck Design
Cover art by Sky Peck Design
Print book interior design by Frame25 Productions
Print book interior images by Shutterstock

Hierophant Publishing
San Antonio, TX
www.hierophantpublishing.com

If you are unable to order this book from your local bookseller, you may order directly from the publisher.

Library of Congress Control Number: 2024951742
ISBN: 978-1-950253-65-4

10 9 8 7 6 5 4 3 2 1

For Josh, Aonghus, and Hamish, and my herbal allies—

you make my world a brighter place.

Contents

Introduction: My Path to Healing   1

Part 1: The World of Plant Spirits

Chapter 1: Rituals of Reconnection   15

Chapter 2: The Sensory Tea Ceremony   29

Chapter 3: The Plant Spirit Journey   41

Chapter 4: Harvesting, Preparing, and Storing Herbs   55

Part II: Plant Spirit Allies for Winter

Chapter 5: Calendula   73

Chapter 6: Dandelion   85

Chapter 7: Rosemary   99

Part III: Plant Spirit Allies for Spring

Chapter 8: Nettle   115

Chapter 9: Cleavers   131

Chapter 10: Wild Oat   143

Part IV: Plant Spirit Allies for Summer

Chapter 11: Hawthorn   159

Chapter 12: Yarrow   175

Chapter 13: Lemon Balm   189

Part V: Plant Spirit Allies for Autumn

Chapter 14: Mullein   205

Chapter 15: Elder   221

Chapter 16: Rose   233

Conclusion: Plant Spirit Allies for Life   249

Acknowledgments   251

Appendix: Opening and Closing Sacred Space   253

Index of Practices   257

Recommended Reading   261

Notes   265

Introduction

My Path to Healing

My path to plant spirit herbalism has been winding, with many stops and detours along the way. I grew up at or below the poverty line, living with my family in several public housing projects. My parents moved us from one side of Scotland to the other and back again, sometimes trying to outrun debts, sometimes trying to find us a better place to live. By age eleven, I had been to five primary schools and lived in nine houses. No matter where we moved, however, there were always two questions at the top of my parents' list when they looked for our next home: Did it have a garden—my dad was a keen gardener—and was it in a rural area?

Because of these frequent moves, I never felt like I fit in with the other kids at school. It was hard for me to make friends, so I retreated into a make-believe world. Fuchsia flowers became ballerinas and I played with them for hours, making them leap and dance. Plants were reliable friends who offered comfort, beauty, and joy without judgment. As I grew older, I realized that working with plants could also teach me a lot about science, a subject that had always fascinated me. When I was seventeen, I decided to enroll in an herbal medicine course at the local university and turn my love of plants into a career.

I spent the next four years immersed in the science of plants, physiology, pathophysiology, and herbal constituents. This suited me well. I loved exploring how things worked, pulling herbs apart and examining them under a microscope. And I loved the fact that we got to wear white coats and stethoscopes and call the people who came to our student clinics "patients."

I certainly had no time for what I considered the "woo-woo" nonsense that some of my older classmates were discussing about herbs—their "energy," their "wisdom," and the "healing" they could offer human beings that had nothing to do with their physical medicinal properties. My parents were fixated on alternative health and spirituality. They were always fussing with crystals and meditation and special diets, and it pleased me to rebel against that by insisting on a more scientific worldview.

After graduation, I opened an herbal medicine clinic where I followed the process I had been taught: work out what's going on with a person and prescribe the appropriate herbs, usually in the form of pills or dried teas that had been packaged in a lab or factory far away. I never gave a thought to the herbs as living beings; they were just resources at my disposal. I certainly never considered the ways in which herbs could provide spiritual guidance and emotional support. I focused strictly on their physical actions.

Over time, I began to yearn for something more than the reductionist, mainstream model of herbal medicine I had been taught. I began to study shamanism (I use this word to refer to the spiritual practices of Indigenous peoples worldwide before the advent of modern religions, not just the Siberian tribe from which the term originated), and realized that I could have a relationship with plants that went far beyond using them to treat physical ailments. Shamanism taught me that herbs are so much more than the compounds we can extract from them. They are wise teachers and loving friends, and when we take the time to connect with them—not just physically, but mentally, emotionally, and spiritually—our lives become much richer for it.

Plant spirit herbalism was born out of my realization that the most powerful healing takes place when we relate to our plant allies on all four of these levels—physical, mental, emotional, and spiritual—rather than simply ingesting capsules, teas, and tinctures hoping they will make us well.

What Is Plant Spirit Herbalism?

Plant spirit herbalism is the practice of engaging with herbs with your whole being, and building relationships with them just as you would with friends. When you meet new people, you don't immediately ask yourself how you can use them or how they can help you. Instead, you get to know them. You pay attention to their personalities, what they like and dislike. You notice the unique qualities that give them their beauty and individuality. Instead of reading about them or stalking them online, you *listen* to them, engaging them in meaningful conversations. And instead of memorizing facts about them—height, weight, blood type— you slowly build shared memories and experiences with them, forging a bond with your heart, not just with your mind.

When we talk about building relationships with people, this direct and intimate approach seems obvious. Yet when it comes to our relationships with plants, we tend to do the opposite. We memorize facts and consult guidebooks, while ignoring the living, breathing entities right in front of us. We focus on their utility, while ignoring their spirits. Imagine how poor our lives would be if we took this attitude with people!

When you practice plant spirit herbalism, plants become living, breathing beings with souls and wisdom. And the more you learn to listen to this wisdom, the more joyful and meaningful your path becomes. Instead of simply learning *about* plants, you learn *from* them. You enter into a co-creative relationship with them, getting to know each one as an individual with unique medicinal properties that go far beyond its well-known physical effects. When you reawaken your five senses, rekindle your imagination, and allow yourself to be guided by intuition rather than book learning alone, you discover what medicine each plant holds for you personally—and this may be very different from what it holds for others.

Plant spirit herbalism is based on two core practices: the sensory tea ceremony and the plant spirit journey. We'll explore both these practices in Part I of this book. They are designed to put you in direct contact with your plant allies and deepen your connection with your sensory self. By tuning in to your senses and using the techniques of meditation, visualization, and sacred ceremony, you can bring your whole self to your relationship with herbs, and uncover guidance and wisdom that is impossible to access when you engage with them only on the material plane.

I have learned many things about myself from using these two practices to communicate with my plant spirit allies, and I share some of these experiences with you in the chapters to come. From hawthorn, I learned how much I tend to be "in my own head," detached from what's happening around me. From yarrow, I discovered that I'm a lot braver than I thought I was. Primrose revealed my tendency to self-isolate when I'm stressed. Indeed, plants can be both mirrors and teachers if we are willing to look. And while what we learn from them may not always be easy or pleasant to acknowledge, treasure awaits us at the end of this path!

Plant spirit herbalism is based on an animist worldview that sees plants as people in their own right, along with rocks, fungi, weather, and mountains. When your perspective shifts into this mode, suddenly everything comes alive. Once you remove the blinders placed on you by modern society—a society that claims humans are the only sentient beings and that everything else is merely an object—you won't be able to put them back on.

And you won't want to, either. When you begin to practice plant spirit herbalism, your world changes from black-and-white to technicolor. Flowers and herbs that used to fade into the background take on vibrant identities and communicate with you in subtle ways. It can take time to fully inhabit this world of spirit—after all, most of us have been taught something very different. But by working with the practices in this book, you can start to welcome deeper meaning, magic, and connection back into your life. You will get to know plants as the individual beings they are—not just as herbs to "use," but as allies you can work with in a reciprocal way.

The Four Medicines Framework

Throughout this book, we will look at herbs through what I call the "four medicines framework," investigating the physical, mental, emotional, and spiritual properties of each plant. This may be a new and unfamiliar concept to many, so let me explain.

- *Physical medicine* relates to the effects herbs have on our bodies—our organs, our bones, and our bodily functions. This is probably the aspect of herbal medicine with which you are most familiar, and the one that has been the most thoroughly documented by science.

- *Mental medicine* relates to the effects herbs have on our cognitive functions, like improving our memory, increasing our focus, and sharpening our mental clarity. Mental medicine also refers to the subtle effects herbs have on our thoughts and our perceptions, and on the attitudes we have toward ourselves and others.

- *Emotional medicine* relates to the effects herbs have on our feelings, our moods, and our emotions. This can take place through the physical effects they have on our nervous and endocrine systems, or through the friendship, guidance, and emotional support they offer.

- *Spiritual medicine* relates to the effects herbs have on a transcendant level—their ability to raise our awareness of our innate connection to the web of life, to awaken a sense of reverence, and to help us access the magic of transformation.

In reality, these healing modalities are not clear-cut. They overlap and merge with one another. In fact, they are not separate, but rather parts of a holistic web of healing that reveals these beautiful plant beings in all their fullness and glory. When you understand how they interact, you begin to bring science and magic back together in your life.

How to Use This Book

Throughout this book, I use the terms "herbal allies" and "plant spirit allies" interchangeably. I encourage you to think of these beings as guides and teachers that can provide you with both healing and wisdom.

In Part I, you will find the tools and concepts that form the foundations of plant spirit herbalism, as well as guidelines for safe and ethical harvesting and instructions for drying and storing herbs. Please read this entire section before moving on to the chapters that follow, because mastering these techniques will ensure your success with the rest of the practices in the book.

Parts II through V focus on herbal allies for each of the four seasons. These chapters contain specific preparations, recipes, and ceremonies for a selection of common plants. You can either read them sequentially or jump to a specific season or herb.

My goal here is not to teach you how to be a medical herbalist. Rather, I aim to teach you how to connect with herbs in a way that allows you to work with the fullness of their medicinal properties in your own life. My best hope is that you will come away with the desire to walk your path surrounded by these compassionate plant beings, some of whom will become your closest allies.

Throughout this book, I encourage you to record your experiences in a journal. Over time, this journal will become a valuable resource for you as you deepen your connection with plant spirits. It will become your very own herbal materia medica that you can consult frequently and expand for the rest of your life.

The herbs discussed in this book are all safe and non-psychoactive. They grow in the world around you. They make their homes in concrete, in gardens, in parks, and in woodlands. What you won't find here are rare and endangered herbs—those that have captured the public imagination and are, as a result, harvested to the verge of extinction.

Plant spirit herbalism is, at its simplest, a hands-in-the-soil, practical methodology. Where possible, I have chosen herbs that are easy to grow and to find. I have provided instructions for making effective herbal preparations for internal and topical use, how to journey to the plant spirit realms for information and healing, and how to conduct ceremonies and rituals for transformation.

Most important, I have attempted to show you ways to access the medicine of plants in a way that is uniquely beneficial to you.

As you walk the path of plant spirit herbalism, you will discover that nature is far richer and more communicative than you ever imagined. You will get to know plant friends and allies that will support you throughout your entire lifetime. And as you do, you will weave a little bit of magic back into your world.

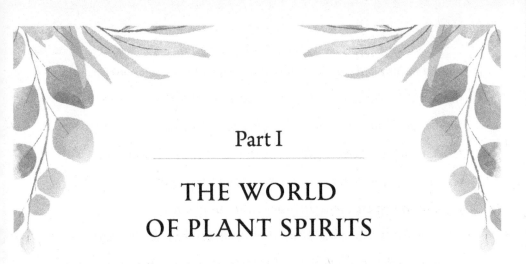

Part I

THE WORLD OF PLANT SPIRITS

Today, we are taught to think about the world of nature rather than experience it directly through our senses. When we see a flower, we reach for an identification guide or open an app on our phones, never pausing to really see, smell, touch, or sense the plant. We read the words on an herbal tea box to learn of its many benefits, then drink the tea without really tasting or appreciating it. We gather information about herbs and think we "know" them—which is a lot like reading someone's online profile and never actually meeting the person.

When asked to describe our friends, we may start with physical features, but we quickly move on to mental, emotional, and even spiritual qualities. Perhaps they are quick-witted or have incredible memories. Perhaps they are prickly with new people, but tenderhearted with those they know and trust. Perhaps there is one special friend to whom we always turn for advice, knowing we will be guided to a state of clarity.

Plant spirit herbalism encourages us to cultivate this same level of relationship with plants. At first, we may describe nettle as a tall green plant with serrated leaves. But when we connect with it on a deeper level, we come to appreciate its personality and uncover the many gifts it holds for us as a teacher and a friend. We recognize it as an ally we can turn to, not just for physical healing, but for advice, comfort, and inspiration.

In order to forge these kinds of relationships, however, we must first reconnect with our own bodies, which are the ground of our awareness. We must regain our ability to truly see, taste, touch, hear, and feel plants—not just in passing, but with our full attention. We can't do this with our thinking minds alone. It requires an embodied sense of connection to the earth and a deep and meaningful relationship with the natural world.

Chapter 1

Rituals of Reconnection

Plant spirit herbalism is based on an intimate, intuitive connection with the natural world. But the society we live in today does not support this kind of connection. In fact, it teaches us to deny and ignore the spiritual dimensions of the world around us and to function solely on a physical and material plane. We are conditioned to doubt our instinctive connection to nature, although we are an integral part of it. We are encouraged to leave behind the world of wonder and imagination we inhabit as children—a world in which we communicate with trees and plants, and converse with animals, and enjoy the company of imaginary friends. We are told to "move on," "grow up," and "get real." In this chapter, we'll explore some techniques that can help you reconnect with this childhood world of wonder so you can begin to develop meaningful relationships with your plant spirit allies.

Hi, I'm Wendy

All good human relationships start with an introduction, and the same is true of your relationships with plants. The first important habit to establish when getting to know a new plant is simply to introduce yourself, just as you would when getting to know a human friend. Once you let a plant know who you are and what you intend, you can begin to form a meaningful connection.

This introduction can be as elaborate or as simple as you like. When a new plant captures my attention or calls out to connect with me, I approach it and say "hello," then tell it my name. I may also make an offering of a small, biodegradable object—flower petals, bread crumbs, or even a strand of my own hair. If time allows, I sit with the plant in a quiet space and soften into hearing whatever wisdom it has to offer. Then I ask it to show me how I can work with it. If I can't spend time with the plant then and there, I visit it later in a plant spirit journey, a practice I describe in detail in chapter 3.

The information that you receive from a plant in your initial meeting can come through in different ways, depending on the plant. Sometimes you hear it; sometimes you sense it, with a kind of inner knowing. Some plants simply enjoy being noticed, and that may be the extent of your reciprocal exchange. Some may become lifelong allies. Others fall somewhere in between.

If the concept of receiving information from plants sounds foreign to you, don't worry. For anyone raised in our materialistic society, this can require a significant shift in perception, and it can take time to feel like you've gotten the hang of it. I often got frustrated early in my shamanic training because I was trying so hard to connect to plant spirits but felt like they were ignoring me. I spent hours sitting with plants, pleading with them to open up and begin a conversation. Sometimes, after many months of trying, I decided that I was done—absolutely no more plant communication for me! But something always drew me back to try again. I don't like to give up easily. When I set my mind to something, I'm "like a dug wae a bone," as the Scottish saying goes—like a dog with the proverbial bone.

One day, as I was listening to a podcast about the importance of using all our senses, I heard something that stopped me in my tracks. We humans forget, a guest pointed out, that there are more ways to communicate than through the spoken word. We also communicate through images, emotions, body language,

RITUALS OF RECONNECTION

and through other subtle cues. Suddenly, the pieces fell into place. I ran outside to sit with a hawthorn tree. I closed my eyes and ears, and opened my heart—and I felt it! I felt the wisdom in my body and the communication in my heart space. I realized that the hawthorn had been communicating with me all along; I just hadn't known how to listen. It was such a relief to know that the plants weren't ignoring me. I was just a slow learner.

Plants communicate primarily through your emotions and through physical sensations in your body. Have you ever looked at a plant and been profoundly moved? Have you ever been captivated by a whiff of beautiful roses wafting on the breeze? Gazed on a sunflower and found yourself smiling? These reactions indicate that the plants are communicating with you; they're saying "hello." And you can increase your chances of catching these subtle messages simply by realizing they are there.

To increase your awareness of these messages, try going for a walk in your local park or in a garden. When you see a plant that is unfamiliar to you, stop and introduce yourself. Tell it your name and where you're from; explain what brings you to the park that day. If possible, make a small offering to the plant, even if it's just a few drops of water from your bottle.

Once you've introduced yourself, pause and pay attention to the plant. Feel deeply into your body, scanning for new sensations or emotions. You may feel warm or cold, tingly or energized, reassured or prickly, joyful or wistful. These are all messages the plant is sending you. Notice them!

When the time feels right to leave, make whatever farewell gesture feels appropriate to you. Return to this plant often and notice how your relationship changes over time.

Attuning to Plant Spirits

Attuning to the spirit of a plant means listening deeply and being open to messages that don't always come in the form you expect. Just as your own body speaks in the form of sensations and intuitions that may not be verbal, plants communicate in subtle ways. As you sit with a plant, images or colors may pop into your head. Old memories may come up, or you may feel waves of emotion or physical sensations like alertness or relaxation. It can be easy to miss these forms of communication if you are lost in hectic thoughts or disconnected from your body.

To attune yourself to the spirits of plants, you must first be attuned to yourself. That means paying close attention to your own physical, mental, emotional, and spiritual state. What is your own body telling you? What is your inner wisdom whispering to you? What is the quality of your awareness? Knowing these things can make it much easier for you to detect the subtle messages of plants.

One way to become more attuned to yourself is to find a quiet spot, sit comfortably, and close your eyes. Breathe deeply through your nose for a count of four. Hold the breath for seven seconds if you are able, then breathe out through your mouth slowly for a count of eight.

With your eyes still closed, shift your attention to your body. Spend a few minutes scanning from your toes to the top of your head, noticing any tension or sensations. Breathe through any areas of discomfort. Don't try to change anything; just notice your body exactly as it is. This will give you a baseline by which to judge any changes that occur. When you are ready, gently open your eyes.

Now go outside and choose a plant on which to focus—a flower, a tree, a shrub, or even the grass. Stand or crouch beside the plant and pay close attention to every detail. How does it smell? How does it look? Are there ants or insects crawling on it? Do its leaves or branches make a sound when they are brushed by the wind?

Pay attention to the sensations in your body. How do your feelings change when you fully engage with the plant? Do you feel a sense of calm? A lift in energy? Any other emotional shifts? Do your sinuses open when you catch its scent? Do your muscles relax? Notice the ways in which engaging with this plant causes you to shift from your baseline.

And remember that you are having an effect on the plant as well. The plant is sensing you just as you are sensing it. You are a part of the plant's environment, just as the plant is a part of yours. How would you like it to feel when it engages with you?

After a few minutes, thank the plant for sharing itself with you. And don't forget to record what you experienced in your journal.

Reconnecting with the Earth

Our planet is a living, breathing organism, and an important part of plant spirit herbalism is reconnecting with the earth under your feet. It is where you come from; it is what sustains you; it is where you will return when all is said and done. Yet we have been taught to think of soil as something unclean. It's no coincidence that it is referred to as "dirt" and looked on as something to avoid.

As a child, I vividly remember the summer days I spent barefoot in the garden. It was tiny, but to me and my siblings, it was a place of magic. There, soil and water became the means of culinary alchemy—no longer just dirt, but chocolate mousse pie that we tried to sell to our younger brother. I also remember the disgust with which we were greeted by adults or older children when our hands were covered in soil and our hair was tangled by the wind. "Get inside; you're disgusting." "Don't play in the dirt; it's gross." Little by little, we learned to avoid touching the earth and to scrub it clean from our feet and fingernails. As we left childhood behind and became more involved in the hectic modern world, we lost our connection to this most fundamental part of our environment.

And yet, that connection is a vital part of your experience. The soles of your feet are rich in nerve endings—over two hundred thousand, according to some estimates. Think of these nerves as your "earthward antennae." When you step on the ground with bare feet or wearing shoes made of thin, natural material, these nerves communicate with the earth and the earth communicates back.

In her seminal book *Women Who Run with Wolves*, Clarissa Pinkola Estés recounts an interaction with a Quiche tribe woman who had gone barefoot until she was in her twenties. When she put on shoes for the first time, she said she felt as if she had blindfolds on her feet. What a vivid picture this paints of just how much we lose when we squeeze our feet into thick-soled rubber and plastic shoes, and go through life never touching the earth at all.

Stepping on the earth barefoot is a deeply spiritual act. Just as a mother and her newborn connect and co-regulate through physical touch, you can ground and replenish yourself by walking barefoot on your earthly home. And this grounded state makes it much easier to focus your attention so you can connect with your plant spirit allies.

Make a practice of walking barefoot whenever it is safe and reasonable to do so, whether in a grassy park, on a beach, or on a gentle forest trail. Notice if walking with your feet in contact with the earth causes you to slow down. Does it heighten your sensitivity to the plants around you? What do you notice that you might not notice otherwise? Do certain plants call to you that you might otherwise overlook? Can you feel the plants' energy more easily when your feet are touching the earth than you would if you were wearing shoes?

Reaching for the Moon

The moon is a stabilizing force for our planet. Without it, the cyclical seasons would disappear and our stable and hospitable environment would become unpredictable and hostile to most life forms—including humans. As the moon revolves around the earth and the earth revolves around the sun, it helps us keep track of time so we can organize and plan. It tells us when it is time to sow and when it is time to reap. These cycles teach us that the passage of time is not linear, but circular. The moon's reflected light teaches us to reflect as well—to pause and consider our actions.

The moon has a profound effect on all aspects of our lives. One study found distinct differences in blood glucose levels and cardiovascular functions in people with type 2 diabetes during different lunar phases.[1] Another large-scale observational study of a million patients over eight years demonstrated that there were noticeable changes in the frequency of outpatient visits to hospitals for fifty-eight different diseases at different points in the lunar cycle.[2] The extra light produced (or more appropriately, reflected) during the Full Moon reduces the amount of melatonin our bodies produce, leading to up to 30 percent less time spent in deep sleep and a reduced amount of sleep overall.[3] In short, our bodies are affected by the moon in ways that we are only beginning to understand.

Just as walking barefoot grounds you and helps you focus, connecting with the moon can heighten your senses and hone your perceptual abilities. It can shift you from a state of abstract thinking to a direct experience of your environment. The more attention you pay to natural cycles, including the lunar cycle, the more you realize that the herbs and plants with which you work are affected by these same cycles. The same moonlight that shines on you is falling on them as well. And this promotes a sense of kinship that is essential to the practice of plant spirit herbalism.

Every Full Moon, make a point of going outdoors and reaching for the moon. Bathe in its beautiful white light. Go to a park or hillside where you can watch the moon rise or set. If you work with sacred objects like crystals, rattles, or drums, this is a perfect opportunity to "charge" them with moonlight.

As you sit and watch the moon, pay close attention to any plants in your environment. Do they also seem to be responding to the moonlight? Have their flowers closed up for the night, or opened wide? Are they releasing scents you don't notice in the daytime? Do they seem calm and sleepy? Or alert and attuned? Do certain plants speak to you more clearly by moonlight than they do in the light of day?

Honoring the Sun

Without the sun, the earth would be lifeless and uninhabitable, and the moon would be dark. Like so many of the forces in our universe, the sun has the capacity to both give and take life. It serves as a time-keeping device and as an aide to navigation. It helps us to heal and supports the cultivation of food. And perhaps most important, it represents the spark of creativity by which all that is formed in the darkness is born into the light.

To understand the spiritual medicine of the sun, we only have to consider its physical effects. Sunlight brings energy and heat. It bleaches clean and removes unwanted substances. It provides illumination and guidance. When you feel lost and unsure of where to go next, or are burdened by the concerns of others, the energy of the sun can help you focus and give you the courage to move forward.

Plants literally eat sunlight. Throughout the cycle of the year, herbs leaf and flower when sunlight is abundant and pull their energy into their roots during the dark of winter. By paying close attention to the power of the sun in your own life, you can better appreciate its role in the lives of your plant spirit allies.

Go out into a park or garden in the early morning and find a comfortable place to sit near some plants, flowers, or trees. As the sun rises, pay close attention to their behavior. Do their flowers or leaves begin to open when the sun appears? Do they stand up straighter? Do their colors change? Do different birds and insects appear? Do certain plants seem happy to see the sun? Do others seem to shrink back, preferring shade? Which plants seem to sing and dance in the light of the sun, and which seem shy and reluctant to speak?

Once you have awakened your senses and restored your connection with the natural world, you are ready to explore the two core practices of plant spirit herbalism—the sensory tea ceremony and the plant spirit journey. The techniques you have learned in this chapter will deepen your experience of both these practices, and unlock ever deeper connections with your plant spirit allies.

Chapter 2

The Sensory Tea Ceremony

As you begin to reconnect with the natural world and deepen your relationship with plants, you will become more sensitive to the unique characteristics and properties of each one. When you get to know individual herbs on a more intimate level, you learn to appreciate the particular flavor each has and what that flavor can tell you about the actions associated with it. This becomes extremely important when performing the sensory tea ceremony, which we will discuss later in this chapter.

The action of an herb refers to its effect on the body, mind, and spirit, and taste can be an important indicator of that action. For example, if an herb tastes salty, or green, that's a clue that it contains minerals that can nourish your nervous system and support your general health. If an herb is strongly aromatic, that often means that it is good for the respiratory system. As you broaden your experience with herbs through practices like the sensory tea ceremony, you begin to develop your own unique knowledge of the actions of your plant allies.

Here is a brief summary of some of the herbal tastes you will encounter, and what actions those tastes may indicate:

- *Bitter herbs* contain compounds called iridoids, alkaloids, and flavonoids that give them their bitter taste. This bitterness is followed by a rush of saliva in the mouth that causes digestive secretions to be released. Bitter herbs can also have a toning effect on the liver and help detoxify the body. Mugwort, turmeric, dandelion, gentian, and motherwort are all examples of bitter herbs.

- *Sour herbs* make you draw in your cheeks a little. They are usually astringent, causing a transient increase of saliva followed by dryness. They often contain compounds called organic acids, like vitamin C and flavonoids, that can reduce inflammation and protect against damage by free radicals. Their astringency can tone weak tissues and is excellent for the liver and the eyes. Examples of sour herbs are raspberry leaf, hibiscus, and rosehips.

- *Salty herbs* are balancing and nourishing. They taste green and grassy, and have a subtle flavor. They are high in minerals like sodium and potassium, and can stimulate lymphatic flow and soften hardened lymph nodes. They tend to support nervous system functions and general well-being. Many are non-irritating diuretics that can nourish and support kidney function. Salty herbs include alfalfa, mullein, nettle, dulse, and kelp.

- *Sweet herbs* tend to be high in carbohydrates, like polysaccharides and saponins. They can build up weakened conditions and low energy reserves. Some common sweet herbs are licorice, astragalus, and Korean ginseng.

- *Spicy and pungent herbs* induce an immediate feeling of warmth. Strongly spicy herbs like cayenne can cause

THE SENSORY TEA CEREMONY

a burning sensation and even pain in the mouth, prompting a rush of saliva that stimulates the digestive system. They often contain compounds called terpenes and iridoids that stimulate the circulatory system and improve blood flow. Spicy herbs have a warming effect on the body and can be helpful for colds and flu. Pungent herbs move energy upward and outward in the body, stimulating digestive secretions, expelling gas, and increasing peristalsis, the muscle movement of the gut associated with bowel movements. Examples of spicy, pungent herbs are cayenne, garlic, and horseradish. Avoid pungent herbs if you are hot, flushed, or irritable.

- *Astringent herbs* leave a dry taste in the mouth that may result in an urge to drink water. They contain tannins, which have a tightening effect on tissues that can reduce inflammation. They can also ease diarrhea and reduce excessive bleeding. They tend to inhibit digestive secretions, so they should be taken between meals. Astringent herbs include witch hazel, rose, yarrow, and oak bark.

- *Mucilaginous herbs* often taste sweet, but their distinguishing feature is their slippery, slimy texture. They have a soothing effect on the mucous membranes and can reduce inflammation. They can also be used to treat coughs and sore throats. Take them with plenty of water, as they are water-loving and can soak it up like a sponge, causing dehydration. Examples of mucilaginous herbs are marshmallow root and slippery elm.

- *Aromatic herbs* taste and smell delightful. They are generally milder in action than pungent herbs, and contain volatile oils called essential oils. They are pleasant-smelling and can stimulate or calm the lungs and nervous system. Many essential oils are antimicrobial and can help fight infections. If taken hot, they can induce perspiration. They also stimulate blood circulation and reduce intestinal gas and spasms. Examples of aromatic herbs are peppermint, lavender, and rosemary.

- *Acrid herbs* taste bitter and burning, a little like bile. Their primary action is antispasmodic, meaning they relax cramps of any kind. Large doses of these herbs often induce vomiting, so they are typically only suitable for use in small amounts for a short time. An intensely acrid herb is lobelia, but milder acrid herbs include vervain and black cohosh.

- *Oily herbs* contain lipids, including fatty acids, which are essential components of cell membranes and necessary for healthy cell functioning. They are also involved in various metabolic processes, including energy production and synthesizing hormones and other signaling molecules. Some essential fatty acids like omega-3 and omega-6 must be consumed, as the body cannot produce them. These herbs tend to leave a slight coating in the mouth. Examples of oily herbs are fennel seed, basil, and oregano.

As you work with the sensory tea ceremony that follows, pay close attention to the taste and action of the herbs you use. This will help you develop an intimate knowledge of your plant allies.

And be sure to take careful notes on what you perceive and experience in your journal. Or, if you like to sketch or paint, use an unlined art book.

Each time you work with a new plant in a sensory tea ceremony, record your experience in words and/or images. Include your impressions of taste, color, and physical effect, as well as mental, emotional, and spiritual qualities. Be sure to include the date and time of the ceremony, as well as whether the herbs you used were fresh or dried. You can even record any dreams you may have. In this way, you build a body of herbal knowledge unique to you.

Sensory Tea Ceremony

The sensory tea ceremony is fundamental to the plant spirit herbalism path. It gives you an opportunity to take a few minutes out of your day and connect mindfully with the tea you are drinking so that you can get to know an herb—its qualities, effects, and spirit—in a very real and tangible way. It's called a *sensory* tea ceremony because it invites you to bring your whole awareness to the act of preparing and drinking an herbal tea, using all of your senses instead of tuning out or giving in to distraction. When you perform this ceremony on a regular basis, you expand your knowledge of herbs beyond their mere physical effects, and learn to appreciate the mental, emotional, and spiritual qualities of each plant.

Think of the last time you drank a cup of herbal tea. Did you notice the fragrance of the rising steam? The shimmering gold, green, or red color of the liquid? Do you remember the subtle emotional and physical shifts you experienced with your very first sip? Did thoughts or memories come into your mind as you drank? Did dreams or wishes make themselves known in your heart? Or were you distracted by your phone or computer screen, relegating the experience of the tea to the background as you clicked, typed, or scrolled?

Perhaps you chose a particular tea for a specific purpose—for instance, helping with indigestion or insomnia. Did you assume that simply gulping down the tea would be enough to resolve your issue? Did you overlook the emotional, mental, and spiritual benefits that can come from forging a deep relationship with the herb? If so, you may have gotten physical benefits from the tea, but you probably missed out on the guidance, comfort, and wisdom that come from honoring the whole plant. This is where the sensory tea ceremony can help.

PLANT SPIRIT HERBALISM

I recommend that you perform this ceremony whenever you work with a new herb. You can also repeat it every time you harvest an herb, deepening your relationship with that herbal ally over time. Every ceremony reveals new layers of subtle awareness. Each time I perform this ceremony with the same herb, I learn new things about the plant spirit and become ever more attuned to it.

The ceremony remains the same for any herb—just follow the steps below for the herb you choose. I recommend using a plain white mug so you can see the color of the tea more clearly. It is best to work with single herbs and avoid adding any extras like honey or milk, as these can alter the flavor and appearance of the tea and result in different effects on your body and mind.

Begin by brewing your herbal tea, paying attention to the aroma released when the boiling water first touches the fresh or dried herbs. Notice how the color changes or deepens the longer it steeps. Take a few deep breaths, inviting the fragrance of the steam to touch your olfactory bulb and enter deep into your lungs. Know that your body is already responding to any volatile oils or compounds contained in the steam. Notice the details. Appreciate the bouquet.

THE SENSORY TEA CEREMONY

State your intention to connect with all the medicines of the herb—physical, mental, emotional, and spiritual. You can say something like: "Dear yarrow, please help me to know you deeply and appreciate your subtle qualities." Then look in your cup and soften your gaze. What colors do you see? Is the water perfectly transparent, or does it have a milky or cloudy quality? Can you see any particles or sediment suspended in the water? What physical and emotional sensations do you feel as you drink in this color?

Gently close your eyes, hold the cup under your nose, and breathe deeply. What do you smell? How does your body respond? Does the scent bring back certain memories or evoke certain emotions? Do you like this aroma, or do you feel hesitant or cautious? Do you detect any notes of sweetness, bitterness, or sourness? What other words would you use to describe the scent?

Now take your first sip. Feel the liquid as it enters your mouth and slides down your throat. Sit for a moment with this feeling. Do you feel any physical, mental, emotional, or spiritual shifts as the tea enters your body? Does the quality of your thoughts change? Do any specific memories arise? Do you have any flashes of insight or intuition? Spend a moment sitting with your eyes closed and tracking how your body and mind change under the influence of the herb you have consumed.

As you drink the tea, pay attention to your mind, your body, and your heart. Remember that the messages you receive from the herb may not come in the form of spoken words. You may feel bodily sensations as the herb makes its way through your system. For example, you may start to feel tingling in your hands and feet if you are working with an herb that supports circulation, or feel pressure in an area with which the herb has an affinity.

If you feel unpleasant physical sensations, this is the plant telling you how it can help you. For example, when I work with peppermint, I often experience a mild and transient nausea that tells me the herb can ease feelings of queasiness. If a certain herb brings up a difficult childhood memory, this can be a sign that it can heal and release trauma. The more often you repeat this ceremony, the more you will be able to identify patterns particular to certain herbs.

When you have finished drinking the tea, record your impressions in your journal. Be as detailed as possible, including physical, mental, emotional, and spiritual experiences. The notes you take now will be very helpful as you continue your journey.

THE SENSORY TEA CEREMONY

Chapter 3

The Plant Spirit Journey

Long before the existence of scientific laboratories in which plants could be examined under microscopes and tested for their compounds and constituents, human beings found ways to learn about the medicinal properties of plants. Shamans played an important role in this process of discovery, journeying to non-ordinary states of consciousness and communicating directly with the spirits of plants in order to receive information about them. It certainly didn't hurt that shamans were deeply attuned to the natural world, and took careful note of which birds, animals, and insects ate certain herbs, as well as the shapes, colors, and scents of plants associated with healing.

Plant spirit herbalism is grounded in this shamanic tradition of engaging plants with the whole self, including the imagination and intuition. One important tool for doing this is the plant spirit journey, which is a form of meditation in which you engage in a creative dialogue with the herb you are getting to know. By engaging in this dialogue, you come into closer relationship with your herbal allies *and* with your innermost self. You open yourself to receiving not just physical healing, but mental, emotional, and spiritual insights that can guide your path and transform your life.

Some of my students ask if these journeying experiences are real or imaginary, and my answer to this question is always an enthusiastic "yes!" Plant spirit journeys take place in your imagination, which is the bridge between your conscious mind and the spiritual realm. They allow you to perceive and interact with plant spirits, even if you understand those spirits to be projections of your own inner wisdom. The truth is that separated consciousness is an illusion. We are always in dialogue with other forms of consciousness whether we realize it or not, and plant spirit journeys are a way of making that basic truth manifest in everyday life.

A Two-Way Street

So what does it mean to connect with the spirit of a plant, and why is this a valuable practice for an herbalist? In other words, why take a plant spirit journey when you can simply enjoy herbs in the form of teas, tinctures, and other medicines?

Plants, like people, thrive in dynamic, reciprocal relationships. Just like people, they want to be seen, appreciated, respected, and known. When you take the time to know a plant, the plant knows you back—and before you know it, your environment is populated with dear friends. This kind of close alliance cannot be forged through book knowledge alone. Think of the deepest, most meaningful conversations you've had with friends. Did they happen when you were seeking factual information, or when you opened your hearts to one another? Plant spirit journeys provide a container in which you can have this type of deep, meaningful exchange with any herb you choose.

Engaging the spirit of a plant means connecting with its most essential qualities—for example, compassion, courage, tenderness, or love. The qualities you encounter may fit a widely recognized pattern, or they may reveal to you an aspect of the plant that is completely unique. The important thing is to stay open to receiving its medicine, and to remember that you can always access this medicine, whether or not you are still in the vicinity of the original plant.

Unlike human beings, who each possess an individual soul, plants in the same species share a single soul. In other words, a dandelion that grows in Edinburgh will have the same spirit as a dandelion growing in New York City. When you go on a plant spirit journey to meet the Spirit of Dandelion, you connect to a universal Dandelion, not to a specific plant that may be growing in the cracks of your sidewalk. This means that, wherever you go in the world, you can access the same medicine by working with other instances of that plant.

It also means that you can connect to the Spirit of Dandelion, or any other herb, whether you are physically present with that plant or not. This can be extremely helpful if you are traveling and cannot access your herbal allies on the physical plane, or if you wish to connect with a rare herb that is not easily found in your area. Plant spirit journeys allow you to access the wisdom and guidance of your plant allies, or to forge relationships with new ones, no matter where you are in the world or what your physical condition may be.

Finally, if you are used to relating to the physical medicine of a plant, while overlooking its mental, emotional, and spiritual medicines, using plant spirit journeys on a regular basis can help you unlock these tremendous and often-overlooked benefits.

These journeys can open up a whole new world of perception, relationship, and experience, and pave the way to health, clarity, and personal growth.

Embarking on a Plant Spirit Journey

Plant spirit journeys should be beautiful, delightful, and meaningful. They shouldn't feel like hard work. With that in mind, you can adapt the journey given here to suit your own tastes, preferences, aesthetics, and spiritual inclinations. If you practice shamanism, you may wish to incorporate drumming or rattling. If you lean more toward silent meditation or prayer, you can cultivate a deep sense of quiet as you connect to the spirit of the plant. The point is not to take on new or unfamiliar spiritual beliefs, but rather to connect with the mental, emotional, and spiritual medicine of plants in a way that feels meaningful to you.

To begin, gather a fresh or dried specimen of the plant whose spirit you wish to meet, or a photograph or drawing of the plant. Create a sacred space in which to conduct your journey. Lay out a beautiful blanket, light incense, or call in the qualities you wish to be present during your journey—for instance, peace, curiosity, or compassion. You may also want to shake a rattle, cleanse your space with a smoke bundle, or make a spontaneous invocation. Be sure to state your intention for the journey and name the specific plant you would like to connect with. For example: "I am seeking insight about my relationship, and I wish to connect with the Spirit of Yarrow."

When you are ready, close your eyes and visualize yourself walking through a long tunnel with a trusted guide by your side. This guide may take the form of a protective being like a human, an animal, or a mythological creature, or it may appear as a ball of light. When you reach the end of the tunnel, emerge into a vibrant, natural landscape filled with plants, animals, waterfalls, and other natural features.

Visualize yourself and your guide arriving at a resting place like a bench or campfire. It is here that you will meet the spirit of the herb. Imagine this plant spirit arriving. What does it look like? How does it move? Does it make a sound? What are the qualities of its presence? What emotions and physical sensations do you feel when it arrives?

It's been my experience that plant spirits rarely show up looking like the actual physical plant forms. They may show up as animals, as nonhuman forms, as human-like beings, or as colors. Or you may just hear a voice—or something else entirely. Don't worry if you don't have a dramatic, cinematic experience. The point is to be willing to listen and learn, and to let yourself be delighted.

However it appears, greet the plant spirit and introduce yourself, then engage in a dialogue. Ask questions and listen for its wisdom. This communication may come as words, images, sensations, or feelings. Allow the plant spirit to share its healing properties, its uses, and any messages it has for you. Be receptive and grateful for its guidance.

When you feel complete, thank the plant and retrace your steps through the tunnel with the help of your guide. When you emerge from the tunnel, return to your physical body. Take a few deep breaths and feel your connection to the earth. Slowly open your eyes.

Close your sacred space in a way that feels meaningful to you—for example, fold up the blanket, extinguish the incense, or say a few words of gratitude or a statement like: "This space is now closed, but blessings continue to flow."

Some people find it difficult or impossible to see images in their minds, and feel disappointed when they cannot visualize their journeys. Others feel more comfortable with passive contemplation than with the more active, creative process of visualization. If either of these cases is true for you, here is an alternative.

THE PLANT SPIRIT JOURNEY

Gather a fresh or dried specimen of the herb (or a photograph or drawing), then open your sacred space and set your intention as described above. Sit still with your eyes open and simply gaze at the herb you chose. As you do so, pay attention to any emotions or sensations that arise. Do you feel warmth or cold? Sadness or excitement? Do you feel a softening in your heart or a sharpening of your intellect?

If thoughts or distractions intrude, simply notice them and let them go, returning your focus to the herb. Continue to sit still, letting the herb's presence saturate your consciousness. What does this herb want you to know about itself? What do you notice in this highly focused state that you never noticed before? When you feel complete, thank the herb for revealing itself to you. Close your space in whatever way feels meaningful to you.

Regardless of which method you use, when the journey is done, take some time to write down your experiences and insights, and any guidance you received in your journal.

Plant Spirit Altars

Once you are performing plant spirit journeys on a regular basis, you may wish to create an altar to focus your intention and act as a visual representation of your practice. An altar provides a sacred space in which you can connect with the spiritual realm, your higher self, and the energies of the natural world. It acts as a focal point for your spiritual practices and rituals—a spiritual workspace, if you will. It's a place where you can make offerings to honor plant spirits, craft medicines, undertake spirit journeys, and sit in quiet meditation. In short, it is a physical space that embodies your spiritual connection with your plant allies.

A plant spirit altar can help deepen your connection with any herb. For example, if you are working with elder, your altar may feature an elder wand, a sketch you did of an elder umbel, a spoon carved from elder wood, or an elderberry tincture you're in the process of steeping. You may also include small items inspired by your plant spirit journey. For example, if the Spirit of Elder showed up for you as a woman in a blue velvet dress and pearls, place a small piece of blue velvet and some seed pearls on your altar. If you work with herbs in the garden, you can also place seeds and other supplies on your altar before bringing them outside.

Building a plant spirit altar is a deeply personal process, and there is no one-size-fits-all approach. Your altar may also change throughout the year, depending on the season and the plant you are working with. Your altar is a reflection of your unique spiritual journey, so feel free to modify it and let it evolve as your practice grows and changes. It can be as simple or as ornate as you are drawn to make it. Elaborate items or complex arrangements do not necessarily lead to better outcomes, however. It's the thought, the care, and the respect you give to the space that matter most.

Over time, working with your altar may allow you to embark on plant spirit journeys more easily. As you repeat the same process each time, the path of connection becomes deeper and more ingrained, and your encounters with plant spirits take on a new quality of clarity and ease.

Select a quiet and dedicated space for your altar. This can be a table, a shelf, or any flat surface. Just make sure that the space is relatively private, somewhere you can sit or stand comfortably during your spiritual work. It should also be out of reach of little hands or animals that like to explore their environment.

Your altar can be indoors or outside. Indoor altars have the advantage of comfort and protection from the elements, but having your altar in your garden or yard can make for beautiful daily rituals, while giving you ample opportunity to reflect on the forces of growth and decay. You may even wish to create two altars—one indoors, and one in your garden where you can leave offerings for plants in their own natural setting.

Place items on your altar that are meaningful to you. Below are some examples to help you get started, but please follow your intuition. You may decide that nothing here resonates with you. That's perfectly fine. Explore the natural world and find objects that call to you.

- *Images or symbols*: Add pictures or symbols that are meaningful to your practice, such as specific plants, deities, or spirit guides.

- *Plant medicines*: Place any dried herbs, tinctures, or other medicines you create on your altar for a certain time before consuming them.

- *Water element*: Include a bowl of water or a seashell to represent the element of water.

- *Earth element*: Include soil, a potted plant, or a small dish of salt or herbs to symbolize the earth element.

- *Fire element*: Use candles to represent the element of fire.

- *Wind element*: Include a feather to represent the element of air.

You can also add any personal items you like—rattles, drums, or objects from your spiritual journeys. On my personal altar, I have a compass, the skull of a sheep that I found on an omen walk, and an incense burner that belonged to my late uncle. You can also leave a space for seasonal offerings.

To ritually activate your altar, cleanse it energetically with a purification rite like rattling, burning incense, or smudging with an herb bundle. As you do so, state your intention:

This plant spirit altar is dedicated to healing, wisdom, and connection. I set my intention to honor and respect the sacred, to seek guidance and clarity, and to walk the path of truth and light that is for my best and highest good at all times.

The saying "tidy house, tidy mind" is true for your altar space and surrounding area as well. Tidy spaces are best, not just for staying organized, but also for invoking spiritual harmony and protection. Your altar should contain only objects you have put there intentionally. Avoid using it as a dumping ground for non-spiritual items. If you place items on your altar that are subject to decay, like dried leaves that crumble, make a regular practice of taking them out to the garden to compost. Every now and then, do a thorough cleaning of your altar, removing everything from it and putting back only those objects that feel necessary in the moment.

Now that you are familiar with the sensory tea ceremony, have taken a plant spirit journey, and created a plant spirit altar, you are ready to engage with plants on all four levels of the medicine they offer—physical, mental, emotional, and spiritual. In the next chapter, we'll explore techniques for harvesting, preparing, and storing herbs with all four of these healing modalities in mind.

Chapter 4

Harvesting, Preparing, and Storing Herbs

There is something incredibly special about growing or foraging for your own herbs, then lovingly drying them and crafting preparations from them. Harvesting herbs requires you to be in touch with the seasons—to know when certain plants fruit and flower, and when their roots are at their best. Certain plants may call out to you as you walk through the woods or wander through the garden, wanting to be noticed or collected. When this happens, it is always magical.

I recommend taking a plant spirit journey before undertaking a serious harvest or creating an herbal medicine. It gives you an opportunity to ask the herb for guidance in its use, as well as permission to harvest it in the first place. Instead of barging into the forest or garden and harvesting plants willy-nilly, it can put you in the proper mindset of restraint, discernment, and reverence. In some cases, you may undertake a journey only to learn that the herb in question does not want to be harvested at that time. Listen to these messages! The respect you pay to the plants will be rewarded down the road.

In addition to being spiritually prepared to harvest herbs, you need to be 100 percent certain that you can recognize the plant you are setting out to harvest. I've seen dandelions confused with nipplewort, and stinging nettle confused with dead nettle. There are many common look-alikes, and some plants in the same family share certain characteristics. The safest way to build confidence in plant identification is to start slowly and make sure of your identification before gathering. If you have grown the herbs yourself, this is much easier than if you hunt for them in the wild, as you can label them when you plant them and observe them at all their life stages.

Safe Harvesting

Perhaps the best advice I can give you for building your harvesting skills is to find a foraging course in your area. This hands-on experience and the support of a seasoned veteran are invaluable.

Invest in a quality identification guide that covers the plants growing in your area. The Collins field guides are of high quality and easy to navigate, and come in pocket-sized editions that are handy for when you're out and about.

I recommend that you not rely on cell phone apps as your primary means of identification. I've used them for some time now, and I've seen them misidentify too many plants to be confident in their accuracy. They work better as a backup to an identification book. If you are unsure of your identification, don't pick the herb! Take some detailed photos so that you can spend some time later researching its features.

And of course, get to know both the edible and medicinal plants *and* the toxic and poisonous ones that grow in your area. This will make you a better forager and help you avoid dangerous mistakes.

Just as important as harvesting safely is harvesting ethically and in a way that respects the sacred spirit of the plants. Here are some tips to ensure that your harvesting meets these requirements:

- Always thank the plant's spirit for providing you with its bounty. You can say a few words

HARVESTING, PREPARING, AND STORING HERBS 57

of gratitude, or leave a small offering like honey, flower petals, or hair.

- Don't pick the first plant you find; make sure the supply is plentiful before you harvest. By doing this, you avoid picking the last plant and ensure that the other beings who rely on that plant don't go without.

- Only harvest what you can use. It is a wonderful feeling when you come upon a large crop of the plant that you are searching for, and you may be inclined to harvest lots of it. Please don't! Consider the spirit of the plant and the other beings who rely on it.

- Know the laws that govern gathering wild plants in your area, and research the plant you are looking for. Is it abundant in the place where you live? Is it scarce or endangered?

- Be 100 percent certain that the plant you are harvesting is the correct one. There are many look-alikes, some of which may be harmful to your health.

- Consider whether the area you are harvesting from is near a road, farm fields, industrial space, or anywhere that weed killer may have been applied. Plants growing in these areas can accumulate heavy metals, waste products, and harmful chemicals.

- Ask yourself if you really need to harvest a plant to connect to its medicine, or if you can connect in a different way—for example, by gazing at it, drawing it, leaving it an offering, or going on a plant spirit journey. Remember, you don't need to pick every plant, every time!

- Have a plan for how you will process the plant *before* you harvest it. Otherwise, you risk wasting the herbs you've gathered, and this is not an ideal foundation on which to base a relationship with the plant.

In some cases, you may receive special instructions for harvesting an herb from a plant spirit journey. For example, the plant may show you that it wants to be harvested on a Full Moon, or that it wants to be sung to as you harvest it. In cases where you receive no special instructions, you can stick to the following general guidelines for how and when to harvest.

- *Belowground parts*: Generally, roots and rhizomes are better collected in autumn or early winter, as the plant's energy has moved back into the roots, where it will remain throughout the winter.

- *Aboveground parts*: These are best gathered in the morning of a dry day, after the dew has dissipated, but before the sun's heat is too intense. On or near a Full Moon is best, as the energetic pull of the moon draws the active parts of the plant out of the roots and up above ground. The heat of the sun can wilt plants and reduce their energy. If you find the plants you want to harvest look listless, then wait until another day to pick them.

- *Bark*: Bark is usually collected from midspring to early summer, when the sap flows freely, although some prefer to harvest bark in autumn. By winter, bark can become more difficult to remove. You can ask the tree or shrub directly what it prefers.

- *Leaves and stems*: Leaves and stems are best collected when young and before the plant flowers, unless you are collecting the whole plant, in which case you should wait until it has just flowered. Choose small or pruned branches rather than the main trunk.

- *Flowers and petals*: Flowers and petals should be collected when in bud or when they have just opened.

- *Berries and fruit*: Berries and fruit are best gathered when just ripe, before the conversion of vegetable acids into sugars and the beginning of fermentation.

Preparing and Storing Herbs

Just as with harvesting plants, you will sometimes receive special instructions for preparing and using an herb from your plant spirit journey. For example, the plant may show you that it wants to be brewed into a fresh tea, or soaked in oil and turned into a topical salve. In other cases, you may simply want to dry the herbs you've gathered to use throughout the year in a variety of different applications. Here are some things to keep in mind as you prepare to use the herbs you have harvested.

Fresh or Dried?

There are benefits to using both fresh and dried herbs. The simplest way to work with herbs is by using them straight from the ground or off the bush—in other words, freshly harvested. Generally speaking, the fresher the plant, the higher the nutritional value, which is important to bear in mind if you are harvesting the herb for its nutritional content, as with nettle, dandelion, and cleavers. These common but powerful herbs are wonderful when added to salads, made into drinks, and cooked into tasty dishes.

On the other hand, drying herbs enables you to use them year-round, not just when they are in season. Properly and carefully dried herbs are wonderful for use as infusions and decoctions; in fact, this is probably the oldest method of preparing herbs for use and storage. The majority of herbs maintain their potency when dried, with some exceptions, like cleavers (*Galium aparine*). When making infused oils, it is important to make sure the herbs are completely dry before you begin, because any excess moisture in the herbs can lead to the growth of mold and bacteria, which can spoil the oil and make it unsafe to use. The exception to this rule is St. John's Wort (*Hypericum perforatum*) and mullein flowers, which should be used fresh to extract the active constituents.

Garbling

Garbling is the process of separating the desired parts of an herb—leaves, flowers, or roots—from the rest of the plant material and discarding impurities and decayed or deteriorated portions of the plant. It's also one of my favorite words! The care and attention you put into garbling can turn a good-quality harvest into a great-quality harvest. On the flip side, careless garbling can result in waste and spoilage.

To garble correctly, carefully remove any brown, spotted, rotten, or discolored parts of the plant, as well as any parts you won't be using. For example, if you're collecting rose petals, discard the leaves and stems. Then dry the parts of the plant you intend to use.

After drying, you can use a screen to garble the herbs again, breaking them down to a uniform size. This will ensure that they cook or steep evenly when you are ready to use them. During this final sorting stage, remove any twigs or stems you may have missed before.

Drying

Your goal in drying herbs is to have them resemble the living plant in color, aroma, and taste to the greatest extent possible.

You must dry your plants as soon after harvesting as possible to minimize deterioration. This is why I recommend having a plan in place for processing your herbs *before* you harvest them. If you dry herbs too quickly using too much heat, they cook and lose potency. On the other hand, if you dry herbs too slowly, they can become moldy.

When you handle herbs gently, you minimize the chance that they will turn pale or brown instead of staying vibrant in color. A classic example of this is plantain (*Plantago major* or *minor*), which must be handled with great delicacy or it will turn brown when dried and be unsuitable for use. Herbs dry best in warm, shaded, well-ventilated spaces. Circulating air is an essential part of the process. Avoid direct sunlight, as this will degrade the herb.

There are two techniques for drying herbs—passive and active. Passive drying involves laying the herbs out on screens or bundling them and hanging them from the ceiling in a warm room with indirect sunlight and plenty of airflow. This method takes patience, but is accessible to everyone. If you live in an area with high humidity levels or low temperatures, however, you may need to invest in a dehydrator.

By contrast, active drying uses a dehydrator to provide the correct temperature and airflow to dry the herbs. This method is often faster than passive drying, and may produce more consistent results. It also allows you to dry herbs when it's rainy or cold outside, which can be a great boon for herbalists in damp climates.

Storing

Light, heat, moisture, and exposure to air can deteriorate dried herbs. I recommend using clean recycled glass jars with wide mouths and tight-fitting lids for storage. Food-safe plastic containers also work, as long as they are stored in a dark place. In the short term, you can even use paper bags. Always store dried herbs away from direct sunlight and heat—a kitchen cupboard is usually a good option.

Once dried, the aboveground parts of plants last for one year. Dried roots last two to three years. Broken, crushed, or powdered herbs lose potency faster than whole, uncut herbs, so it is best to powder or chop your herbs just before using them.

It is crucial that you properly sterilize glass jars and lids to ensure the safety and longevity of your herbal preparations. You can either boil the jars in water or place them in the oven at 135°C (275°F) for fifteen minutes.

Herbal Preparations

In the following sections of this book, you will find recipes, practices, and rituals that use a number of different herbal preparations. Although I've listed known contraindications for every plant, you should always do your own research about interactions with any medications you are taking, and consult a skilled herbal practitioner for dosage recommendations based on your weight and age, and any health conditions you may have.

Here is an overview of the types of preparations you will find in the chapters that follow.

Tinctures

Tinctures are solutions prepared from fresh or dried plant material combined with alcohol or an alcohol/water blend. Various alcohols are used, including wine, brandy, vodka, and ethyl alcohol, sometimes called Everclear (190 proof/95 percent), or high-grade neutral spirits. For home herbalists, brandy and vodka are the best options. Just be sure the alcohol you use is not flavored with anything.

Tinctures are stable and extremely long-lasting, with a history of use stretching back thousands of years. It is one of the most common forms of herbal medicine used by medical herbalists, as alcohol extracts the widest range of active constituents from the herb. When it comes to tincture dosage, less is more—a couple of drops go a long way.

Infusions

Infusions (sometimes called *tisanes*) are beverages made by steeping fresh or dried herbs in hot or cold water. You can use a single herb or a combination of them. This preparation method uses water to extract the beneficial ingredients and flavors of the plants. A properly prepared infusion is not just a cup of tea—although it looks like one!

Infusions can be hot or cold, depending on the herb. They can be made from fresh, dried, or powdered herbs. Some active constituents are not released easily into water and need longer infusion time or decoction (see below). Be sure to cover pleasant and strong-smelling herbs when infusing them to avoid losing their therapeutic volatile oils in the steam. Most infusions last for up to two days if refrigerated.

Decoctions

Decoction is a traditional method of preparing medicinal teas using tough plant materials like roots, bark, seeds, nuts, and woody stems. In this process, the plant material is gently simmered in water for an extended period of time to extract the beneficial compounds and nutrients. The resulting liquid is then strained and consumed as a therapeutic drink.

Like infusions, decoctions can contain one herb or a combination of them. They are best made fresh, but can be kept in the refrigerator for up to two days. If you are using dried herbs, coarsely grind or thinly slice them before simmering. If you are using fresh herbs, thinly slice roots, shave off small pieces of bark or wood, lightly crush seeds, and roughly chop leaves and whole herbs.

Syrups and Electuaries

A syrup is a water extract of an herb that is then preserved with a sweetener, typically honey or sugar. Electuaries are made from finely powdered herbs mixed with honey. They can vary in consistency from a runny liquid to a thick paste, depending on how much herb is blended with the honey. They are useful for anyone who cannot (or will not) tolerate strong flavors or bitter herbs.

Glycerites

Glycerites are made by extracting the active ingredients from herbs using glycerin—a liquid whose action falls somewhere between alcohol and water. These extracts offer a unique approach to harnessing the therapeutic properties of herbs, distinct from traditional alcohol-based tinctures or water-based decoctions. They provide a gentle and versatile means of extracting herbal constituents, particularly tannins and volatile oils, but are not suitable for use with herbs that have a high resin or gum content, like myrrh.

Glycerin tastes sweet, but does not impact blood sugar or yeast levels. It has antiseptic and soothing properties when diluted with water. You can mix glycerites with water, alcoholic extracts, vinegar extracts, or any combination of these. They appeal to individuals seeking alcohol-free remedies or more palatable herbal formulations, and are a great option for children. They are, however, more expensive to make than tinctures and don't extract quite as broad a range of constituents. Nonetheless, for certain herbs, they are worth considering.

Topical Applications

The human body can absorb herbal compounds through the skin, and topical applications are a useful alternative for those who cannot or will not tolerate internal remedies. They also work well as an adjunct to internal herbal remedies, treating from both the inside and the outside. Topical applications range from simple baths and compresses to ointments, salves, and poultices.

No matter which type of herbal preparation you use, remember to connect with the herb on all four levels of medicine: physical, mental, emotional, and spiritual. How do you feel as you harvest, garble, and process the plant? What are the nature and quality of your thoughts as you extract the herb's active constituents? How do you perceive the herb guiding you? What are your hopes for how this plant will heal you? As you experiment with these preparations, return to your plant spirit altar frequently to meditate, journey, and connect with your plant allies in ways that feel meaningful to you.

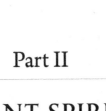

Part II

PLANT SPIRIT ALLIES FOR WINTER

Winter is an in-between time. It is a waiting period full of possibilities yet unknown, and it can be hard to wait for those possibilities to peek up over the horizon. We are rarely content to be in a state of contemplation, slow unfolding, and eventual transformation. We want things to happen now. But winter, with her chilly fingers, counsels patience.

Winter is a time to be still and bask in pure potential. In the darkness of the season, we can set aside our masks and any ideas we may have about who we are. From this position of surrender, we can make space for the gradual unfolding of what comes next, without forcing it or imposing our own ideas on it. We can rest in the darkness, giving our souls room to breathe and gathering energy for the spring to come.

In the deep stillness of winter, we counteract the darkness by feasting. As we increase our intake of sugars, fats, and, in many cases, alcohol, our digestive systems suffer. The pleasure we take in our winter feasts is often counterbalanced by swollen bellies and loudly voiced regrets. In many parts of the world, cold temperatures reduce circulation and aggravate aching bones. Increased dryness worsens skin and sinus conditions. All this encourages us to hibernate indoors and exercise less. And this reduction in activity reduces the flow of lymph, which further impacts our health.

Herbal allies for winter can help us settle into this season of deep contemplation, while gently supporting the health challenges it brings. Cheerful, warming, and steady, they remind us that the return of the sun is just over the horizon, and that the best things in life are worth waiting for.

Chapter 5

Calendula

Common names: *calendula, pot marigold*
Latin name: *Calendula officinalis*
Family: *Asteraceae/Compositae*
Parts used: *whole flower heads, including green calyx*

Calendula is one of my original herbal allies. This flower was among the first to welcome me enthusiastically when I began my plant spirit herbalism journey, and one of the first herbs I successfully grew in my garden. It was forgiving, surviving animal interference, the rough touch of young children, and my own bumbling attempts to nurture it. It thrived and bloomed until the first frost. Its Latin name is derived from *calends,* which fell on the first day of every month in the Roman calendar. This references its extended flowering season.

The Spirit of Calendula was a light in the darkness for me when I was in the middle of what felt like a storm—a time when almost everything I had known before was stripped away and I hadn't yet found my safe harbor. Its bright flowers shone like a lighthouse for me, one that I could see from my bedroom window when I woke in the morning to give me the courage to get up and move, and one that I could wish goodnight as I closed my eyes and welcomed the escape of sleep.

Many have described calendula as a light in the darkness, and I certainly found this to be true. In her wonderful reference book *A Modern Herbal*, Maud Grieve writes:

> [Calendula] has been cultivated in the kitchen garden for the flowers, which are dried for broth, and said to comfort the heart and spirits.[1]

With its support for the digestive and lymphatic systems, calendula is the perfect herb for the dark winter months. I like to harvest and dry a nice supply of these flowers to use throughout the winter in infusions, sitz baths, and rituals.

Habitat

Calendula is native to many areas, including mainland Europe, the Middle East, North Africa, and Western and Central Asia. In North America and the UK, it is most often found in gardens, but it can also appear as an escapee, blooming in meadows and fields. These adaptable plants grow in various soil types, but perform best in loamy or sandy soil, in full sun to partial shade. They prefer temperate climates and can tolerate mild frost, but not extreme heat or cold.

Identification

Calendula is like a ray of sunshine. These bright, daisy-like flowers can grow up to 60 cm (2') tall in colors ranging from bright yellow to deep orange. The blossoms have a central disc surrounded by ray florets. Each is about 4–7 cm (1½–3") in diameter, and the underside green calyx is sticky to the touch. The leaves are oblong and slightly paddle-shaped, and are arranged in an alternate pattern along the stem. The leaves and stems are pale to bright green and slightly hairy.

Harvesting, Drying, and Storing

When newly opened, the whole flower heads of calendula are ready to harvest. When you feel underneath where the petals join the rest of the flower, the green calyx should be slightly sticky to the touch. This sticky, resinous compound is an important part of its medicine. You can collect the flower heads right through the growing season and the plant will continue to blossom. In milder years, I have had calendula flowering from June until November. Harvest on a dry and sunny day, as this plant tends to hold on to moisture and can be tricky to dry. Snip the entire flower head off using secateurs, removing as little of the stem as possible.

Calendula flowers can be dried passively or in a dehydrator set to 40°C (104°F) for eleven to twelve hours. If you are drying more than one tray of flower heads, swap the trays every few hours to ensure even drying. They can take twenty-four to thirty-six hours to dry if the weather is wet before harvest.

Over time, your dried calendula flowers will lose their vibrant color. But as long as they still have their characteristic scent, they retain their medicinal benefit.

Contraindications

Avoid calendula during pregnancy or if you have any known allergies to the daisy family.

Four Sacred Medicines

In the Introduction, we talked briefly about what I call the "four medicines framework," which outlines the physical, mental, emotional, and spiritual properties of each plant. In the chapters that follow, we'll look at how each of these four healing modalities are manifested in the actions of individual herbs.

Physical Medicine

Calendula is a versatile herb used in many different types of preparations to treat a broad range of medical conditions.

- *Skin conditions*: Calendula is a primary wound healer and is my go-to herb for skin healing, especially when there is redness, inflammation, pus, and heat present in the wound. It acts on a deep level by increasing circulation and lymph flow to the area.

- *Bleeding*: Calendula helps stop bleeding and encourages wound healing by supporting angiogenesis, the repair of damaged blood vessels. It also increases collagen production to close and heal wounds.[2] For wound healing, working both externally and internally with calendula yields the best results.

- *Lymphatic system*: Calendula wakes up a slow or struggling lymph system, as it improves both the flow and clearing capacity. It is a valuable addition whenever lymphatic support is required, when chronic hard or swollen glands are present, or when fluid retention or oedema is an issue.

- *Digestive tract*: Calendula's impact on the digestive tract begins in the mouth. You can use a calendula infusion as a twice-daily mouthwash to treat bleeding gums or infection.[3]

- *Mucous membranes*: Calendula can be used to treat any pain or inflammation in the mucous membrane that lines the digestive tract, as in ulcers, Crohn's disease, and inflammatory bowel disorders.

- *Digestive lining*: Calendula can heal and restore the integrity of the digestive lining, as in leaky gut syndrome.[4] Its bitter properties gently stimulate digestion, which is beneficial for sluggish digestion linked to inflammation. This results in a healthy combination of digestive stimulation and mucous membrane healing.

I like to use calendula when food intolerance is an issue and when chronic digestive problems like bloating, constipation, or indigestion are present—especially when hard or swollen lymph glands are a factor. Digestive issues can also show up as skin conditions, bad breath, and an increase in body odor as the body struggles to eliminate waste via the usual channels.

Mental Medicine

If you are sensitive to changes in seasons, especially when summer days make way for longer nights in autumn and winter, calendula can be like a ray of sunshine that can help you navigate this tricky time. Calendula lifts and supports. It is not a magic bullet that can remove the sadness or discomfort you may feel during the winter months; it is more like a trusted friend that will walk your path with you and help you make sense of your experience.

Emotional Medicine

The physical medicine of calendula points to its emotional action—wound healing. If you are dealing with trauma that has been repressed and closed off while you focused on survival, calendula can support the process of revelation, transformation, and release. The heavy, steady nature of its resins also supports the integration of new patterns and behaviors. Of course, it is always wise to address these issues with the help of a trusted therapist.

Spiritual Medicine

The spiritual medicine of calendula is like a beacon in the darkness, revealing truth and insight that has been hidden from the conscious mind. If you are looking for clarity or insight into a particular situation or problem, calendula can help. It acts like a piercing ray of sunshine on a foggy winter day that cuts through the mist to reveal the landscape beyond, making visible what was hidden.

In plant spirit journeys, calendula often shows up as a deeply protective plant, guarding your physical, mental, emotional, and spiritual boundaries against energetic intrusions. If you are feeling stuck and stagnant, unable to move forward, or unsure of which direction to take, calendula's gentle and persistent heat stokes your inner pilot light and encourages you to begin moving again.

Working with Calendula

Here are three ways you can work with calendula to achieve physical and spiritual healing.

Practice: Hot Calendula Flower Infusion

You can drink this hot infusion to lift your spirits and support your physical health during the cold months of winter or at any time of the year.

Just pour about 250ml (1 cup) of boiling water over 10–15g (½ oz.) of chopped dried calendula flowers and stir well. Let stand for ten to twenty minutes, then strain and enjoy warm.

Practice: Healing Calendula Sitz Bath

Sitz baths are warm, shallow baths used to relieve pain and discomfort in the genital area. They are particularly suited to healing after childbirth, pelvic pain associated with ovulation or menstruation, and conditions like hemorrhoids and anal fissures.

For this sitz bath, make 500ml (2 cups) of a strong calendula infusion as described above using 50g (2 oz.) of dried herbs and 500ml (2 cups) of boiling water. Fill a large basin with warm water and add the herbal infusion. When the water reaches a comfortable temperature, sit in it for fifteen to twenty minutes. Add extra hot water as required. You can use calendula alone, or add other herbs such as yarrow and lavender. You can enjoy sitz baths up to three times daily.

Practice: Calendula Healing Ceremony

In this ceremony, you work with both the physical medicine of calendula and the spirit of the plant to support you during the dark winter months.

You will need:

- Calendula flower infusion (see above)

- A quiet and comfortable space to sit or lie down

- A blanket

- Your journal and a pen to record your experience

Begin by purifying yourself and your space in a way that feels meaningful to you. Open your space in your usual way, remembering to call in the Spirit of Calendula.

Start with a sensory tea ceremony (see chapter 2), slowly drinking the calendula infusion and attuning to your physical and

82   PLANT SPIRIT HERBALISM

emotional responses to the herb. When you have finished drinking the infusion, lie down and cover yourself with the blanket.

Imagine the sunny brightness of the calendula flower coming into your body, igniting your inner pilot light, and giving you the strength you need to make it through the winter. You may visualize this light as yellow, orange, or gold in color. It may appear as a small flicker or a full flame. However tiny it may be, however, know that this light will always be there for you.

As you lie still, allow any insights or messages to come through from the Spirit of Calendula. When you feel complete, close the ceremony in a way that feels meaningful to you, and record your experience in your journal.

Chapter 6

Dandelion

Common name: *dandelion*
Latin name: *Taraxacum officinalis*
Family: *Asteraceae/Compositae*
Parts used: *roots, leaves, flowers, and seed pods*

Gardeners have long considered dandelions a nuisance. I suspect this is part of their appeal for me—the inner rebel rejoicing in a bit of chaos. But dandelions are actually quite useful. Their deep taproots provide nutrients for the plants around them and loosen compacted soil. Like the equally maligned dock plant, they aerate the soil and help reduce erosion. They come into their own as they cleanse and support the beings and the land where they grow, improving conditions for all other plants and wildlife around them. The magic of dandelion lies in its practical, gentle, and intentional transformation of anything with which it comes into contact.

Dandelion medicine came to me after an exhausting school holiday. It was a time of sadness, as the kids were returning to school, but also a time of relief. I love my children deeply, but looking after their differing needs during the school holidays is tiring! My husband and I had little time together and were knocking heads on an issue we couldn't get past. We decided to have a last picnic on the front lawn, which was alight with the liquid sunshine of dandelion flowers. After we ate, the children went off to explore.

I lay down among the flowers, closed my eyes, and felt the deeply restorative energy of dandelion wash over me. It was palpable and so enjoyable. In just a few moments, the answer to the problem we had been wrestling with came to me clearly. When I opened my eyes, my husband and I had a deep and heartfelt conversation, supported by the Spirit of Dandelion.

Dandelion's bright yellow flowers open with the first morning light and close again in the evening, highlighting its strong affinity with the sun and its power to get things moving. It is one of the first flowers to bloom in spring and among the last to go dormant in winter. Dandelions are an important early source of nectar and pollen for bees, and their seed pods provide delight for all ages.

Habitat

Native to Asia and mainland Europe, dandelion is now found throughout the world. It grows almost anywhere, but is common in cultivated areas and wastelands. It also thrives in rich meadows, pastures, and fields.

Identification

The smooth, hairless or sparsely haired leaves of this plant can grow from 5–50 cm (2–20") long and 2–10 cm (1–4") wide. They are deeply toothed, giving them a jagged or "lion's tooth" appearance. In fact, this plant's name derives from the French *dent de lion*, meaning "lion's tooth." The leaves form a basal rosette, meaning they grow in a circular pattern from the base of the plant, close to the ground.

Each flower grows on a single, hollow stem that is usually leafless and can be 5–60 cm (2–24") tall. They are bright yellow and composed of numerous tiny petals. After flowering, dandelions form spherical seed heads known as "puffballs" that are white and fluffy, and look like a Full Moon.

Be aware that there are similar-looking plants, like wild lettuce or sow thistle, that can be mistaken for dandelions. Dandelions are distinguished by their single flower per stem and lack of branching.

Harvesting, Drying, and Storing

Harvest dandelion parts from spring through autumn. For the roots, unearth the plant and trim the leaves to dry separately. Wash and chop the roots into roughly even pieces about the size of a pinky finger. If you only harvest the leaves, trim them from the plant and the dandelion will continue to grow.

Dandelion roots can be dried passively or using a dehydrator set to 43°C (110°F) for twelve to twenty-four hours. Roots are dry when they snap cleanly. The leaves can be dried passively or using a dehydrator set to 38°C (100°F) for twelve hours or overnight.

Contraindications

Avoid dandelion if you have an allergy to the daisy family, or if you suffer from a closure of bile ducts and cholecystitis.

Dandelion leaf is a very effective diuretic, so caution should be taken if you are taking prescription diuretics.

Four Sacred Medicines

Here's how dandelion fits into the four medicines framework. Note its varied physical, mental, emotional, and spiritual properties, and how they are manifested in the medicinal actions of the plant.

Physical Medicine

Dandelion acts primarily on the digestive system and is useful in mantaining blood sugar levels and fighting inflammation.

- *Digestive system*: Dandelion root has an affinity with the liver and digestive tract. It encourages the production of digestive enzymes and supports gut bacteria in its many tasks. As a result, it is helpful in any conditions where digestion is sluggish, like constipation, bloating, and excessive burping or flatulence. Consider using dandelion roots for conditions driven by poor liver and digestive function, like PMS, menstrual cycle irregularities, and polycystic ovarian syndrome (PCOS). It can also be used to treat chronic skin conditions like acne, eczema, and dermatitis.

- *Blood sugar*: The slightly sweet taste of dandelion root indicates that it is beneficial in balancing blood sugar levels. It can support those who tend to feel tired after eating and crave sweet or salty foods. It can also play a vital supportive role in type 2 diabetes or metabolic syndrome.

- *Inflammation*: When used topically as an infused oil, dandelion flowers are anti-inflammatory and can benefit joint pain and inflammation. They combine well with daisies and comfrey leaf in a topical infused-oil treatment for acute sprain, strain-type injuries, or muscle soreness that comes from a heavy workout. The flowers are particularly indicated if tension is a contributing factor.

Mental Medicine

If you feel lonely, isolated, deeply fearful, detached, or dissociated, dandelion connects you to yourself, your authentic nature, and the web of life, helping bring forth your inner warrior. Working with dandelion can often bring about a welcome release of fear and tears. The flowers are wonderful at gently breaking you free from a blocked space when your creativity has dried up and you feel uninspired and listless.

Emotional Medicine

Dandelion can help if you are experiencing anger, bitterness, and resentment that you are unable to let go, especially if the anger is turned inward. It can also help you get to the deep root of an issue, which is perfect if you need clarity about what is happening.

Spiritual Medicine

Dandelions are like the sun; if you feel blocked, especially creatively, they bring vitality, energy, warmth, and determination. In plant spirit journeys, they often show up to connect you to spiritual messages you may have been unable to hear due to disconnection, self-doubt, or distrust of your body.

Working with Dandelion

Here are three practices that draw upon the Spirit of Dandelion.

Practice: Dandelion Root Tincture

Dandelion root tincture is ideal for use in the winter months to counteract the heavier food choices and occasional over-indulgence associated with this time of year. I recommend twenty to thirty drops prior to eating to help your digestive system.

Sterilize and dry a large glass jar with a lid that can be tightly closed. Fill the jar one-third to one-half full with dried, chopped dandelion root. Add enough brandy or vodka to completely cover the herbs, leaving a small gap between the top of the liquid and the lid to account for expansion of the herb. Make sure that all of the plant parts are covered.

Cap the jar tightly, shake well for a minute or so, and store it in a dark, dry place. Check after twelve hours to see if the herb has absorbed all the alcohol. If it has, add more until the herb is covered again. Shake the jar daily (or as often as you remember) for four weeks.

After four weeks (or a lunar cycle), pour the tincture through a muslin- or cheesecloth-lined strainer into a jug and squeeze as much of the liquid out of the herbs as you can. Bottle, cap, and label the finished tincture and store it out of direct sunlight in a cool place. Put the spent herbs out on your compost heap.

Practice: Italian Dandelion Soup (Cicoria)

A student of mine once proudly shared this story and recipe with me. One day, out of the blue, her grandmother called her and started talking about dandelions. They had had no prior conversations about this plant, but her grandmother knew she was studying herbs. This conversation led to unearthing a family recipe that had been passed down through generations. It also created a new bond that reached back through history.

To make this soup, you will need:

- 1 bunch dandelion greens

- 1 medium sweet onion

- 60ml (¼ cup) sundried tomatoes

- 1 shallot

- 3 cloves garlic

- 3 tablespoons olive oil

- 1 liter (4 cups) chicken or vegetable stock

- Salt and pepper

- Red pepper flakes to taste

Optional garnishes include fresh parsley, fresh lemon juice, grated pecorino romano, or grated Parmesan.

Wash and chop the dandelion, dice the onion, julienne the sundried tomatoes, and mince the shallot and garlic. Place the olive oil, onion, tomatoes, and shallot in a stock pot and sauté on medium heat until translucent. Add minced garlic to the mixture and cook until fragrant.

Pour the stock over the vegetable blend and simmer for ten minutes. Add the dandelion greens and simmer until wilted. Garnish with red pepper flakes, a squeeze of fresh lemon juice, and a sprinkle of cheese, and enjoy!

Practice: Dandelion Herbal Amulet

An herbal amulet is a small, wearable charm made from plants or plant materials—roots, berries, bark, nuts, etc. It serves as a tangible connection to the plant spirit and harnesses the sacred medicines of the plant to support the wearer on all levels.

Plants are not only sources of physical remedies, but also powerful allies in spiritual work. Carrying or wearing an herbal amulet invokes a plant's guidance, protection, and healing in daily life. You can adapt the ceremony below for any herb or combination of herbs you like.

To make this amulet, you will need:

- A quiet space where you will not be disturbed

- A dried dandelion root (large enough to carve a hole in)

- A small knife or carving tool

- A length of string or cord (preferably natural fiber) sufficient to make a small necklace

- A natural beeswax candle and lighter or matches

Before you begin, decide which aspect of dandelion medicine you want to manifest—for example, grounding or resilience.

Cleanse yourself and open your space in your usual way, remembering to call in the spirit medicine of dandelion. Sit comfortably and close your eyes. Take some slow, deep breaths, then visualize roots extending from your feet into the earth, anchoring you firmly. Feel the stability and support of Mother Earth beneath you. Open your eyes and state your intention:

DANDELION

95

*I call upon the Spirit of Dandelion to guide and protect
me in a way that is for my best and highest good. This
amulet embodies the sacred medicine I choose to invoke.*

Light the candle and spend some time reflecting on which of the dandelion's sacred medicines you wish to embody with your amulet.

When you feel ready, pick up the dandelion root and carving tool. Carefully carve a hole through the center of the root. Thread the string or cord through the hole and tie the ends in a knot. You can charge the amulet by holding it over the candle flame (at a safe distance) and saying:

*By the power of fire, I charge this amulet
with the strength and clarity of my intention.*

Place the amulet around your neck and sit quietly as you feel into the properties of the plant. When you are finished, thank the dandelion and any other helpful, compassionate spirits you invoked. Snuff out the candle to close the ritual space, saying:

This space is now closed, but my connection
to dandelion continues and blessings flow.

Wear your dandelion amulet for as long as you are guided—a few days, a few weeks, or longer. When you take it off, you can place it on your altar to use again. Or you can return it to nature, ideally near the place where it was harvested. This closes the circle and lets the plant return to the earth.

Chapter 7

Rosemary

Common names: *rosemary, polar plant, compass weed*
Latin names: *Rosmarinus officinalis, Salvia rosmarinus*
Family: *Lamiaceae*
Parts used: *aerial parts, leaves, soft stem tops*

Rosemary, also known as the friendship bush or the plant of friendship, is one of my dearest herbal allies. I work with it daily, using a dried bundle to smoke cleanse my space before starting my working day. I inhale its scent later in the day when my brain is foggy and I'm struggling to concentrate. I find rosemary's steady and enduring quality both deeply comforting and uplifting. I love nothing more than gently stroking rosemary leaves and inhaling the fresh, pine-like scent. Rosemary brings warmth to the colder winter months and is deeply protective at this time of death and renewal.

The botanical name for rosemary, *Rosmarinus officinalis,* comes from the Latin words *ros,* meaning "dew," and *marinus,* meaning "of the sea." This name may reflect rosemary's native habitat along the Mediterranean coast. I just love this name, and I can imagine the green leaves of the plant glittering with sea spray as the sun rises high overhead—a reminder that brighter days are coming.

Habitat

Native to the Mediterranean, rosemary thrives in climates characterized by warm, dry summers and mild, wet winters. It grows best in well-drained, sandy, or loamy soils, and thrives in coastal regions, rocky hillsides, and dry scrub.

This hardy shrub thrives in these arid environments because it can withstand drought conditions and poor soil quality. While it flourishes in full sunlight, it can tolerate partial shade. Its resilience and adaptability allow it to grow in many settings, but it thrives in places that mimic its native Mediterranean home.

Identification

Rosemary is a perennial shrub that usually grows to about 1 m (3½') in height, but can reach up to 2 m (6½'). The leaves are linear, about 1 cm (½") long, and resemble small curved pine needles. They are dark green and shiny on top, with a white underside and curled leaf margins. The small bluish flowers grow in axillary clusters (at the base of the leaves), and the plant has a delightful and unmistakable aroma.

Harvesting, Drying, and Storing

You can harvest small amounts of the leaves and soft stems of rosemary throughout the summer months. For a larger harvest, you can combine this with a yearly pruning of the bush. Make sure you cut with sharp secateurs to avoid damaging the stem that's left behind. Take the upper portions of the shoots with the leaves on, and strip off the leaves from the portions of the shoots that are very woody.

You can dry rosemary passively by hanging small bunches of stems and leaves upside down in a dry, dark, warm, and well-ventilated space, or use a dehydrator set to 35°C (96°F) for seven to nine hours.

When completely dry, the leaves should still smell strongly of rosemary, but will be brittle and crumbly. If the stems are woody, strip the leaves from them and either place them on your compost heap or store them for use as skewers for cooking vegetables or meat.

Contraindications

Avoid using rosemary essential oil during pregnancy or if trying to conceive. Be cautious about using it if you are taking iron supplements, as research shows it inhibits iron absorption.[1]

Four Sacred Medicines

Rosemary combines all four of the sacred medicines into one powerful healing herb.

Physical Medicine

Rosemary is one of the most versatile herbs for physical healing.

- *Anti-inflammatory and immune support*: Rosemary has strong antioxidant benefits from constituents like rosmarinic and carnosic acids.[2] Antioxidants help protect cells from damage caused by free radicals.

Normal metabolism produces free radicals as a by-product, but they also come from pollution, radiation, and smoking.

- *Antioxidant support*: Our bodies are designed to cope with a small amount of free radicals, but too many can damage cells, proteins, and DNA, ultimately leading to diseases like cancer and heart conditions. Rosemary's antioxidant action also reduces inflammation and supports immune health.

- *Digestive and respiratory systems*: Research has shown that rosemary may heal the mucosal lining of the digestive tract, especially where ulceration has occurred.[3] It soothes the smooth muscle that lines the digestive and respiratory tracts, easing digestive issues like gas, bloating, and cramping. It is also effective for treating respiratory conditions caused by narrow airways, like asthma and COPD.

- *Antimicrobial support*: Research backs up what traditional herbalists have long known—that rosemary has strong antimicrobial properties.[4] Its extracts can

ROSEMARY

inhibit the growth of many types of bacteria, including *Escherichia coli, Staphylococcus aureus*, and *Salmonella typhimurium*. It also has demonstrated antifungal properties against *Candida albicans*, a common cause of fungal infections.[5] This action works both internally and topically. Whenever infection and inflammation are present, rosemary is a great choice.

- *Circulation*: Rosemary can be beneficial when circulation is poor—think cold hands and feet, Raynaud's syndrome, varicose veins, or tinnitus and vertigo. It can help manage fevers because it warms and supports the circulatory system, moving blood from the body's core to the skin and allowing heat to disperse through the pores.

- *Post-viral depletion and chronic stress*: If you feel exhausted and depleted after an infection or a long period of stress, rosemary supports your nervous and immune systems.

Mental Medicine

If you are feeling scattered, foggy-headed, or unsure where you are in life, rosemary can help you recalibrate so that your path becomes clearer and you can start moving forward again. Like pouring a small amount of fuel on a dying fire, it gives you a burst of energy. If you are feeling down—if your mental chatter is focused on the negative or on things you are doing wrong— it uplifts you and gently shifts your perspective just enough so that you can begin connecting with the small glimmers of joy and gratitude that have been hidden.

Rosemary has long been known as an herb of remembrance, and research is now showing that it supports mental alertness and memory. In a randomized controlled trial, rosemary essential oil was shown to decrease frontal alpha and beta power, which leads to more focused task engagement.[6] In other words, it helps you focus and keeps you focused. During exams at university, I carried this deeply supportive herb to help me concentrate.

Emotional Medicine

Because it is an herb that supports the nervous system, rosemary brings you back to yourself when you are disconnected or disassociated due to long-term stress and trauma. It can relight your inner fire when you've been carrying a heavy mental load and are struggling to connect with inner joy and purpose.

Spiritual Medicine

If you are undergoing change or upheaval, rosemary can walk by your side as a steady, protective ally. This herb is very cleansing on all levels. If you have had a difficult interaction or have been out and about in public, it can cleanse and ground you. It can protect you if you are entering into a tricky or unpleasant experience or if you tend to get overwhelmed in busy, crowded places. It is one of my favorite bodyguards, along with yarrow and nettle.

Rosemary draws energy up and out, and connects you with your intuition and the spirit realm. With its support, you hear spirit messages more clearly and put them into action more easily. If you doubt your intuitive abilities or are actively working to hone them, rosemary is an excellent ally.

Working with Rosemary

Here are two simple practices that can help you harness the power of this plant spirit ally.

Practice: Rosemary and Sage Infused Wine

Although not as commonly used these days, wine's combination of water and alcohol effectively extracts a wide range of herbal constituents. The antioxidants in wine, like resveratrol, are an added medicinal benefit. The alcohol acts as a natural preservative and extends the life of your preparation. Wine can also improve the taste of herbal extracts, making them more enjoyable.

This recipe was inspired by *The Herball, or Generall Historie of Plantes* by John Gerard, which was first published in 1597. To prepare it, you will need:

- 250ml (1 cup) dried rosemary leaves

- 250ml (1 cup) dried sage leaves

- 750ml (1 bottle) dry white wine

Ensure the herbs have been dried thoroughly to prevent mold and spoilage, then place them in a sterilized glass jar or large glass bottle. Pour the wine over the herbs until they are completely covered and the jar or bottle is filled, leaving a little space at the top. Seal the jar or bottle tightly with a lid or cork.

Place the container in a cool, dark place and let it infuse for two weeks. Shake it gently every few days to mix the contents. After two weeks, strain the wine through a fine mesh sieve or cheesecloth into a clean glass bottle. Squeeze out as much liquid as possible from the herbs for maximum benefit. Label the bottle clearly with the date and contents, then store it in a cool, dark place.

Take a small glass of the infused wine as a tonic to improve memory and overall vitality. This preparation was historically consumed in moderation as part of a health regimen—rosemary for its ability to strengthen memory and improve overall health, and sage for its support of the nerves and longevity.

Practice: Rosemary Smoke-Cleansing Ceremony

Indigenous cultures around the world have practiced smoke cleansing for millennia. This ritual involves using the smoke of burning herbs, woods, and resins to purify a space and make it sacred. Smoke cleansing supports focused intentions, deep connection, and spiritual exploration. It can help create a shield of spiritual protection to ensure a safe and sacred environment. In this ceremony, we will use dried rosemary.

Please note that animals (particularly birds) do not do well with smoke, so make sure that your space is free of pets. Avoid smoke cleansing when pregnant and when around young children. Check with your healthcare practitioner if you have a pre-existing respiratory condition. And always make sure that your smoke bundle or loose herb mix is completely extinguished when you are finished. Never leave a smoke bundle unattended.

Once lit, loose and bundled herbs will generally smoke for a minute or so, and you can relight them as required. If you want more copious smoke, you can use a charcoal disc. I recommend doing this outdoors or in a well-ventilated room, as it can be a very intense experience.

Begin by clarifying your intention. Reflect on what you want to cleanse or release. Gather a bundle of dried rosemary stalks or put some loose leaves into a heat-resistant container. Carefully ignite the bundle's tip or the loose herb using matches or a lighter. Allow the flames to catch, then blow them out, letting the herb smolder and release its fragrant smoke. If you are working with a bundle, hold it over a heat-resistant container to catch any embers that may fall.

Begin at the entry point of the space you're cleansing, then move clockwise throughout the area, fanning the smoke with a feather or your hand. If you are cleansing your body, begin at

ROSEMARY

your head and work down the front of your body, then repeat the process at your back.

As you move, recite your intention or affirmation. Visualize the smoke as a purifying force, dispelling negativity and imbuing the space with positive energy. Relight the bundle or loose herb as necessary.

When you are done, gently extinguish the bundle by pressing it into the heat-resistant container. If you are using a loose herb, wait until the smoke subsides and make sure it's completely out before storing it. Thank the spirits for their assistance in your cleansing journey.

Of course, rosemary is not the only herb you can use to smoke cleanse. Just be sure to do your research to confirm that the plant you are burning is not toxic. Here are some favorites:

- *Juniper (leaf and branches):* Juniper is known for its deeply protective properties against negative energies, spirits, or influences, as well as its refreshing and invigorating characteristics. Juniper smoke can clear the mind, reduce mental clutter, and promote clarity. It is often used to prepare for meditation or introspection.

- *Mint and lemon balm*: Use this blend if you are tired or need a fresh perspective. Lemon balm brings calm, relaxation, and emotional balance; mint brings freshness, vitality, and rejuvenation.

- *Mugwort (aboveground parts)*: Mugwort is useful for opening ceremonial spaces, deciphering metaphorical messages from plant spirit journeys, and enhancing dream work. This creative and contemplative plant is also very grounding.

- *Pine resin and pine needles*: Pine is a cleansing, protective, and grounding herb, useful if you're feeling a little out of your body after a ceremony or plant spirit journey. Pine resin is very protective; just think of the role it plays in protecting a wounded tree trunk.

- *Rose petals*: Smoke cleansing with rose can give you courage and clarity, as the thorns are symbolic of piercing the veil or cutting through to the heart of the matter. Rose can also help you uphold energetic boundaries.

- *Rowan (berries, leaf, and wood)*: Smoke cleansing with rowan berries can clear the mind, reduce stress, and enhance mental focus. The leaves and branches have a rich history of providing spiritual protection and warding off negative energies.

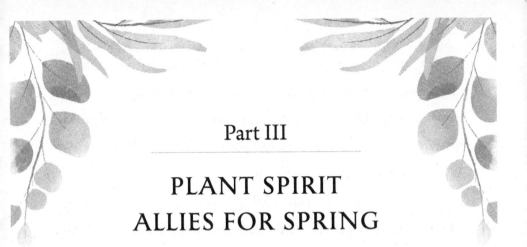

Part III

PLANT SPIRIT ALLIES FOR SPRING

Spring is a transitional time when winter and summer push and pull, the dance of warm days alternating with sudden cold snaps. As nature awakens from its slumber, the dreams we gestated in the dark of winter begin to push their way through into reality. This causes us to pause and reflect. Are we on the right path? Are there changes we can make so that the seeds we sow will bloom into our soul-aligned purpose? Do we need to weed out anything that is not serving us?

The trees wait until a certain number of warm days have passed before trusting that it is indeed spring and not a false warm spell. Then they experience an awakening. In early spring, before leaves unfurl, their equivalent of our eyes—the transparent covering of their buds—perceive changes in light and trigger a set of responses that prepare them to meet the coming season.[1] Their sap starts to rise, providing the nutrients and water required for growth.

The hypothalamus—a structure deep in our brains—prompts a similar awakening. It begins to respond to the slow increase in daylight, initiating responses that impact our appetite, our sleep patterns, and parts of our immune system. This signals our pineal glands to produce slightly lower levels of melatonin, the sleep hormone, and we begin to wake up earlier.

As trees begin to flower, seasonal allergies make an appearance, putting our immune systems at risk. As the days grow longer, our adrenal glands begin to produce slightly more cortisol. The early-morning production of this stress hormone prompts a response that contributes to a sense of increased energy. This helps our state of mind, but shuts down our digestive functions.

Our herbal allies for spring help us meet the challenges we encounter as our bodies seek balance and rejuvenation. Their spirits encourage us to be more like the trees—our sap rising, our new leaves unfurling, our souls ready to embrace the next steps on our path.

Chapter 8

Nettle

Common names: *nettle, stinging nettle*

Latin name: *Urtica dioica*

Family: *Urticaceae*

Parts used: *young leaves collected before flowering, roots collected in late autumn, seeds collected in mid- to late summer*

The Scottish poet Thomas Campbell very accurately described the varied uses of nettle:

> In Scotland I have eaten nettles, I have slept in nettle sheets and have dined off a nettle table cloth. The stalks of the old nettle are as good as flax for making cloth.[1]

Nettle is one of Scotland's most valued plants. Indeed, an alternative name for May Day is Nettlemass Night because, on the evening before the Celtic festival of Beltaine, people drank a cleansing preparation of the plant. Nettle is high in protein and also contains large quantities of minerals, including iron. In their own way, our Celtic ancestors were both purifying themselves—nettle is a deeply cleansing herb—and providing their bodies with the building blocks required to meet the increasing busyness of the season.

Although nettle flowers are small and not particularly showy, this plant has always commanded my attention. It's not one of the first spring plants to arrive, but when I spot those jagged leaves, I rejoice at their return. Sometimes the bundles of seeds have an almost purple hue and, when they are backlit by the sun, they take on an otherworldly air as they sway slowly back and forth in the breeze.

Nettle seeds are adaptogens—plants that help support and protect the body against stress. You may be more familiar with more exotic adaptogens like ginseng, ashwaganda, and holy basil. But nettle grows everywhere—and is not endangered. With a few tools and a bit of patience, you can harvest and dry the seeds. And then it's dealers' choice—you can put them in smoothies, bake

116   PLANT SPIRIT HERBALISM

them into cookies, grind them slightly and add them to a tea blend, or make a tincture and take a few drops daily. They dry easily and store well, and the added bonus of their nutritional content is another compelling reason to make nettle a part of your diet.

I love the Latin name for nettle—*Urtica*, meaning "to burn"—because it is so descriptive of the pain that accompanies the nettle's sting. Another name for the plant is *dioica*, which means "of two houses." And in fact, nettle is one of only 5 percent of flowering plants that have male and female flowers on separate plants; the rest have male and female parts on the same plant.

When I am preparing nettle leaves and seeds for drying, I wear cotton gloves, although I prefer using my bare hands for garbling and drying. My fingers can tingle for days after, and I enjoy this reminder of the potency of nettle's medicine!

While the medicinal power of this plant is strongest in young leaves harvested before flowering, you can also cut back nettle during and after flowering and use the regrowth later in the summer. Be aware, however, that older leaves are unsuitable for medicinal purposes as they contain cystoliths that irritate the urinary tract.

NETTLE

Habitat

Nettle is found in many parts of the world, including North America, Europe, Asia, and parts of Africa. Its habitat can be quite diverse, as it can adapt to different environmental conditions. Generally speaking, it prefers partial to full shade and likes to keep its feet damp (it loves to grow near water). It can also be found as a pioneer species on disturbed, cultivated ground. This perennial lives for over two years, spreading through underground rhizomes and forming dense colonies.

Identification

Seventeenth-century herbalist Nicholas Culpeper observed that nettle is "so well-known that they need no description at all, they may be found by feeling around in the darkest night."[2] And in fact, nettle is one of the more easily identified plants.

Nettle leaves grow opposite each other on the stem and have a serrated margin (toothed edges). They are heart-shaped with a pointed tip and have a slightly rough texture. The leaves are green and can grow up to several centimeters (2–3") in length. These plants can vary in height, typically reaching 60–120 cm (2–4') tall. But they can grow even taller under favorable conditions. Their stems are square—a characteristic shared by the mint and vervain families.

In summer, nettle plants produce small, inconspicuous greenish or brownish flowers that are arranged in elongated clusters. The female plants then produce abundant green seeds, which are held on little strings that hang down underneath the leaves.

Perhaps the most distinctive feature of nettle is the presence of tiny, needle-like hairs on the leaves and stems. These hairs contain chemicals like formic acid and histamine that cause a stinging sensation. There are some similar-looking plants, like dead nettle (white or purple), but while these look as if they bite, their leaves have no sting—an excellent way to differentiate!

Harvesting, Drying, and Storing

To harvest nettle leaves, snip the stem approximately 15 cm (6") from the base or above the point where the leaves look old, worn, or eaten by insects. In early spring, you can dry both the tender stems and leaves for use. By late spring and early summer, you can snip the whole stem again, remove the individual leaves, and put the fibrous stalks on your compost heap.

Dry nettle leaves and stems passively or with a dehydrator set to 42°C (107°F) for twelve hours or overnight. To harvest nettle

NETTLE   119

seeds, snip the stem just below the last bunch of seeds. Leave these spread out outside for a few hours to let any insects escape. Then snip off the individual strings of seeds and lay them flat on trays. Dry the seeds passively or with a dehydrator set to 42°C (107°F) for twelve hours or overnight.

If using nettle seeds for teas or tinctures, you can leave them on the strings and store them in an airtight container. If you are using them for baking or in your cooking, remove them from the strings by rubbing them gently between your fingers over a bowl. Put the fibrous strings on your compost heap. Once dried, nettle leaves and seeds last for a year. The dried root lasts two to three years.

Contraindications

This is a safe and well-tolerated herb with no known contraindications for use with medications or during pregnancy or lactation. Of course, avoid using it if you have a nettle allergy.

Four Sacred Medicines

Nettle is one of the most versatile herbs, with applications across all four of the sacred healing modalities.

Physical Medicine

The internationally renowned herbalist David Hoffmann once said: "If in doubt, give nettles." I tend to agree with this. Nettle is a generous herb that really gets the job done! Its leaves are nutritious, and it has a wide range of applications as a medicine.

- *Skin conditions*: As a strong alterative and anti-inflammatory, nettle can treat skin conditions like eczema and dermatitis, especially when there is an element of anxiety driving or worsening the issue.

- *Allergies*: For conditions like hay fever and allergic rhinitis, nettle has an anti-inflammatory effect. It also regulates the immune reaction and lessens the production of histamine, which is the primary cause of sneezing, watery eyes, and runny nose. For this, nettle combines really well in an herbal tea with equal parts elderflower (*Sambucus nigra*) and plantain (*Plantago major/minor*).

- *Intestinal tract*: As a drying and astringent herb, nettle is effective in treating chronic diarrhea and mucus in the stool. This action also makes it useful in treating internal and external bleeding like nose-bleeds, cuts and wounds, bleeding hemorrhoids, and heavy menstrual periods. For this, it combines well with yarrow (*achillea millefolium*).

- *Urinary tract*: Nettle has an affinity for the urinary tract, especially when there is the kind of pain and inflammation you might experience with kidney stones or an active infection. Try making a tea with equal parts nettle leaf, corn silk, and heather to help soothe and heal.

- *Postpartum care*: Nettle is deeply supportive and nutritive, and especially beneficial when you are exhausted and depleted. It's a wonderful herb to use for postpartum care and beyond, particularly if you are breastfeeding. For this, it combines well with fennel seed as a tea.

- *Anemia*: Nettle can help to replenish iron levels and is helpful in anemia associated with heavy periods. In addition, its astringent nature can help to lighten heavy periods.

- *Prostate support*: Nettle root is mainly used for enlarged prostate conditions, particularly benign prostate hyperplasia (BPH). By reducing the activity of sex hormone-binding globulin (SHBG) in the prostate, it can alleviate symptoms and restore zest for life.

- *Kidneys and adrenal glands*: Nettle seed has an affinity for the kidneys and the adrenal glands. It can also help those struggling with poor kidney function, or the loss of a kidney.

Nettle is very nutritious and is a good source of vitamins A, C, E, F, K, and P, as well as zinc, magnesium, iron, copper, selenium, boron, bromine, chlorine, chlorophyll, potassium, phosphorus, sodium, silica, iodine, chromium, silicon, and sulphur. It also provides high levels of calcium and vitamin B complexes. I prescribe nettle seed when someone is feeling low on energy and vitality, or wakes up feeling tired and wanting to go back to bed. I drink nettle seed tea most days upon waking, and I find it gently stimulating and nourishing. In other words, it makes for a lovely start to my day.

Mental Medicine

Nettle balances your inner mental landscape and helps you move out of stagnation. If you are feeling stuck and unmotivated, it can wake you up and clear your path for forward movement. Likewise, if your mind is working at a million miles an hour, it can slow you down so you can become more present and reconnect with your body and your intuition.

Like yarrow, nettle can help you find your courage when you are faced with a task that you really want to do, but can't seem to summon the strength to accomplish.

Emotional Medicine

This deeply caring and nourishing plant connects you to your inner fire and resilience, moving you out of a state of apathy or emotional stasis. Nettle encourages you to stand tall, to bend with the breeze, and to go after what you cherish the most. Its affinity with water and the kidneys makes it a useful ally when you are working on issues with relationships and communication.

Spiritual Medicine

Nettle is a wise elder in plant form. Strong and fierce, it often shows up in plant spirit journeys to help you hold your boundaries when you have difficulty standing your ground. It can also support work with ancestral issues. Its strong fibers help reweave the strands of broken or damaged ancestral connections and help to remove curses, particularly those that run down generations of family.

Working with Nettle

Here are two delicious recipes made with nettle. Try them as you prepare for the cleansing and renewal ceremony at the end of the chapter.

Practice: Nettle Leaf Pesto

Young nettle leaves are a nutritional spring treat that can be frozen for use throughout the rest of the year when the plant is too old to harvest or has died back for the winter. If you love to forage and have wild garlic or leek growing near you, you can substitute these for the nettles.

To prepare this recipe, you will need:

- 500ml (2 cups) young nettle leaves (wear gloves to handle)

- 120ml (½ cup) fresh basil leaves

NETTLE   125

- 120ml (½ cup) grated Parmesan cheese (for a vegan option, try 60ml (¼ cup) of nutritional yeast)

- 120ml (½ cup) pine nuts (you can substitute walnuts or almonds)

- 3 garlic cloves

- 120ml (½ cup) extra virgin olive oil

- 1 tablespoon lemon juice

- Salt and pepper to taste

Bring a pot of water to a boil. Using gloves or tongs, add the nettle leaves and blanch them for about one minute, then transfer them to a bowl of ice water to stop the cooking process. Drain the leaves and squeeze out any excess water.

In a food processor, combine the blanched nettle leaves, basil, Parmesan cheese (or nutritional yeast), pine nuts, and garlic cloves. Pulse the mixture until it is finely chopped. With the food processor running, slowly pour in the olive oil. Blend until the mixture is smooth and creamy. Add the lemon juice and season to taste with salt and pepper. Blend again to combine all the ingredients.

Transfer the pesto to a jar or bowl. It can be stored in the refrigerator for up to a week. For longer storage, spoon it into ice cube trays and freeze until solid, then transfer the frozen cubes to a freezer-safe bag or container. The pesto will last in the freezer for up to six months. To use, just thaw the desired amount in the refrigerator or at room temperature.

Practice: Spring Greens Vinegar

I like to make this herbal vinegar at the beginning of the growth season for the mineral-rich herbs. It never lasts me long enough, despite the fact that I make more each year—a testament to how delicious it is. You can use nettle alone, or combine it with other herbs in any ratio you like.

To prepare this, you will need:

- A sterilized glass jar with a lid

- Waxed parchment paper to stop the vinegar from corroding the metal lid

- Apple cider vinegar

- Fresh and washed spring herb leaves—dandelion, nettle, hawthorn, plantain, wild raspberry, cleavers, or wild violet

NETTLE 127

Finely chop the herbs and place them in the sterilized glass jar. Pour apple cider vinegar over the top until the jar is filled almost to the top. Place parchment paper over the opening and screw the lid down tightly.

Place the jar in a dark place and shake it daily, or as often as you remember. Strain the mixture after two weeks and label the jar with the date, the names of the herbs, and the type of vinegar. Then enjoy this mineral-rich condiment. I like to put a half teaspoon of it in my drinking water to start my day. It also makes a delicious salad dressing.

Put the discarded leaves on your compost heap.

Practice: Nettle Ceremony for Cleansing and Renewal

This herb's spirit medicine cleanses and renews as you prepare for the dreams of winter to manifest. Perform this ceremony whenever you feel stuck, stagnant, or in need of rejuvenation. All you need is a quiet, undisturbed space and some nettle leaf infusion.

Start by infusing two teaspoons of chopped, dried nettle leaves in 200ml (1 cup) of hot water for at least fifteen minutes. Then strain the leaves and pour the infusion into a cup to use in the ceremony.

Cleanse yourself and open your space in your usual way, remembering to call in the Spirit of Nettle. Sit comfortably and close your eyes. Take deep breaths and feel your connection to the earth beneath you. Place your hands on your heart and state your intention for the ceremony:

Nettle strengthens and rejuvenates me, removing the
remnants of winter and infusing me with the vitality of spring.

Open your eyes and hold the cup of nettle leaf infusion in your hands. Take a moment to look at the color and to breathe in the green aliveness. Take a deep breath of the steam and savor the aroma. Slowly drink the infusion, feeling its warmth and vitality entering your body. With each sip, visualize the infusion cleansing you physically, removing toxins and revitalizing your cells.

Imagine this physical cleansing spreading to all levels of your being—clarifying your mind, purifying your emotions, and uplifting your spirit. Feel the renewal flowing through you, clearing away any stagnant energies or blockages.

Once you have finished drinking the infusion, stand up and begin a series of gentle, flowing movements. Start by raising your arms to the sky, drawing down the energy of the sun. Then slowly lower them and shower yourself with light. Begin to move your body in a way that feels good to you—twisting, stretching, swaying. Let your body lead the way. Let go of any notions about what you "should" be doing. Move to release; move to embrace; move to step fully into spring. Remember, whatever you release is transmuted into loving compost for the earth.

When you feel complete, thank the Spirit of Nettle for its presence and wisdom. Sit quietly for a few moments, reflecting on the ceremony and any insights or messages you received. Allow the energies of cleansing and renewal to integrate fully into your being. Close your sacred space in your usual way.

Following the ceremony, gift the remaining nettle leaves back to the earth. They make wonderful compost!

Chapter 9

Cleavers

Common names: *cleavers, goosegrass, lady's bedstraw*
Latin name: *Galium aparine*
Family: *Rubiaceae (bedstraw family)*
Parts used: *aerial parts harvested in spring before the seeds form*

If you were allowed to roam free in the countryside as a child, you are probably familiar with cleavers—a scraggly, scrambling, weak-stemmed plant that clings to your clothes like Velcro. Because its leaves, stems, and seeds are covered in tiny hooks, it sticks to just about anything, and many parents have spent long hours despairing over cleavers tangled in their children's hair and clothing. In Britain in the early twentieth century, if cleavers were thrown and stuck to a girl's back without her noticing, it meant she had a sweetheart. If she pulled them off and dropped them on the ground, they were said to form the initials of her sweetheart-to-be.

When I was a child, my siblings and I had hours of fun throwing handfuls of cleavers at each other to see if they stuck. We also made little dolls from the stems, which are easy to bend and weave. And cleavers were among the first plant spirit allies I encountered when I started my transition from a strictly scientific and materialistic worldview to one that made space for a little more intuition. The woven stems of this plant were traditionally used to strain unwanted contaminants from milk; in a similar fashion, they helped me filter and strain my ideas so I could gain a clear vision of how to weave my new way of being in the world.

Cleavers' Latin name is *Galium aparine*, with *aparine* being Greek for "to seize"—a fitting name for a plant that grabs you and holds on! Some of its other names point to it being a very practical plant. Dried and matted cleavers were once used to fill mattresses, hence the name bedstraw. Another common name, goosegrass, calls to mind the animal that most enjoys its juicy green stems—although many other animals relish this tasty herb as well.

In fact, this herb comes complete with a sense of adventure, resilience, and playfulness, making it a wonderful companion to keep by your side in the spring.

Habitat

Cleavers is an abundant plant found in many diverse environments. Naturally widespread in Europe, the UK, North America, and some parts of Asia, it has been introduced as far south as Australia and New Zealand. It pops up in hedges, scrub, open woodlands, waste ground, and shingle beaches, and sometimes even makes its presence known in cultivated ground and among crops.

Identification

Cleavers are undisciplined, climbing annuals with a very distinct four-angled square stem—similar to the type found in the mint family. They can grow from 50–200 cm (20–80") tall and are covered in minute, down-curved prickles like tiny hooks. The leaves are narrow and oblong with a pointed tip, and are arranged in patterns of six to nine whorls around the stem. Like the stem, they are also covered in small, hooked bristles. These do not hurt to touch, but are prickly enough to grab on to passing animals—an excellent strategy for seed dispersal.

The tiny flowers are white and funnel-shaped, with four spreading petal lobes. From these come the round two-lobed seeds, which are also covered in hooked bristles.

Harvesting, Drying, and Storing

Cleavers do not survive the drying process particularly well, so I recommend harvesting this plant in the spring, before the seeds appear. You can make a tincture from the fresh plant, but this requires a high-proof alcohol like Everclear, which can be tricky to find if you live outside of the United States. In the UK, you need a license to purchase liquor of this strength, and for this you need to be a registered herbal practitioner or manufacturer.

I prefer the simplicity of working with cleavers fresh, either in hot infusions or cold overnight infusions. To use these infusions throughout the year, freeze them in ice-cube trays and defrost as needed.

Be aware that, despite their rambling, rambunctious nature, cleavers have a shallow root system, so harvest plants gently to avoid pulling them out by the roots.

Contraindications

This herb has no known contraindications. Cleavers is a gentle diuretic, however, so be sure to drink plenty of water to counteract potential dehydration.

Four Sacred Medicines

The Spirit of Cleavers has properties that make it an effective ally when working with all four of the sacred medicines.

Physical Medicine

Cleavers physical medicine relates primarily to the urinary tract and the lymphatic system.

- *Urinary tract*: As a diuretic, this herb supports urinary functions, as in the case of bladder infections. It can help your body flush out excessive fluids and salts.

- *Lymphatic system:* This is one of the few herbs that support the lymphatic system. It can help get the lymph moving again, removing any lingering waste from the system. Due to its high water content, this plant works best as a short-term remedy when it is at its peak in spring. Some of the key signs that the lymphatic system needs support include swollen glands or recurring tonsillitis, skin outbreaks, fluid retention, sore and tender breasts before menstrual periods, and feeling tired, lethargic, and unmotivated.

Mental Medicine

If you tend to get tunnel vision or find yourself agonizing over a project's details, this plant's rambling, spreading nature helps you move forward step-by-step, covering more ground than you thought possible. Its sticky nature can give you the tenacity you need to stay with a tricky problem until the solution reveals itself to you.

Emotional Medicine

If you feel emotionally cluttered to the point of being overwhelmed, cleavers can give you the courage, energy, and motivation to begin clearing things out. Its playfulness can help you release tension if you take yourself too seriously, and remind you that there are sweet days—and possible sweethearts—still to come.

Spiritual Medicine

In a plant spirit journey, this herb often shows up to help you set healthy boundaries in relationships, especially when there are messy entanglements and enmeshments involved—just think of the tangled mess into which this rambling plant grows!

This energetic and curious herb also shows up when you yearn for adventure, but have a list of excuses that keep you safe. Its spirit helps you move out of a state of disconnection, stagnation, and unhappiness, and into one of spontaneity and joy.

Working with Cleavers

These three practices bring the substantial powers of this herb to your aid wherever and whenever you need help.

Practice: Spring Cleansing Infusion

I like to drink a cold infusion of cleavers every day in the spring, when this gregarious plant is at its best. This cleansing beverage gets your lymph flowing and encourages your winter-weary spirit to come out of hibernation and play.

To make this infusion, you will need:

- A handful of cleavers (young, springtime shoots)

- Enough cold spring water to cover the herb completely

- A sterilized glass jar with a lid

- 2 or 3 slices of fresh lemon (optional)

Wash and roughly chop the cleavers and put them in the glass jar with the lemon (if you are using it), then add spring water. Cap the jar tightly and place it in the refrigerator for at least six to eight hours or overnight. Strain the mixture and enjoy your cleansing drink.

Practice: Cleavers Coffee

Making this coffee substitute is labor-intensive, but it is worth the effort for the late-summer pick-me-up it can give you. Enlist some energetic children to help you pick the seeds! Also, be aware that these seeds are *extremely* hard when dried, so you'll need a good seed or coffee grinder.

Gather at least 100g (3½ oz.) of dry, brown cleavers seeds by picking them off the stems and then discarding the stems. Preheat the oven to 180°C (350°F). Place the seeds on a baking tray and dry roast them for forty-five minutes to an hour. The more seeds you have, the longer the roasting will take.

Let the seeds roast until they smell like weak coffee and have turned a little darker, but don't let them burn. When they are ready, remove the seeds from the oven and allow them to cool slightly before grinding them. Or you can store them for later use and grind them as needed. Add one teaspoon of ground seeds to a mug of fresh water, infuse it for fifteen minutes, and strain. Then enjoy the fruits of your labor.

If you like the flavor of cardamom (I adore it!), try adding half a cardamom pod when infusing. This has the added benefit of supporting your digestive system.

Practice: Cleavers Talisman Ceremony

Springtime brings a sense of adventure. But for some of us, this is a difficult energy to embrace. This talisman-crafting ceremony focuses on releasing emotional and mental blocks that inhibit your sense of adventure. The word *talisman* comes from the Greek word *telesma*, which means "to consecrate and fulfill." Talismans thus help fulfill a desire or intention in a sacred way. They are traditionally crafted from animal, vegetable, or mineral ingredients, and range from very simple to extremely elaborate.

Talismans are usually created in a ritual setting that focuses thoughts or intentions in such a way that they either live in the talisman or come to a state of completion when the talisman is destroyed. They can also be created as offerings to deities, gods and goddesses, or nature spirits. They can be burned, buried, or taken apart for release and healing. Or they can be kept to amplify an intention and attract benefits and protection.

Remember that this is not a beauty contest. Put aside any thoughts of how you want your talisman to look. Work on this sacred object in an intuitive way. It may end up looking like a bundle of sticks wrapped in twine, but that doesn't affect its purpose and power.

To make this talisman, you will need:

- A small handful of fresh cleavers

- A candle

- A quiet and sacred space to carry out the ceremony

- Background music to play while crafting the talisman

Gather your supplies and open your space in your usual way, remembering to call in the spirit medicine of cleavers. Then play your music and light the candle.

Before you begin to craft, call to mind your intention. Is there something specific you want to do, but are reluctant to try? What would it look like if you said "yes" and leaned into the potential outcome? When you feel ready, speak your intention aloud:

The talisman I am about to craft with the blessing
of cleavers connects me to my sense of adventure.

Slowly begin crafting, knowing that the intention you hold will also be held in the talisman. As you work, pay attention to how the plant material feels in your hands. You may decide to weave the cleavers into a mat, or form them into any shape you like. You'll find that they stick together well and that you won't need extra bindings.

When you are finished, charge the talisman by holding it over the candle flame at a safe distance and saying:

By the power of fire, I charge this talisman
with the strength and clarity of my intention.

CLEAVERS

Place the talisman on your plant spirit altar and close your space by snuffing out the candle and saying:

I give my thanks to cleavers. Blessings
continue to flow and this space is now closed.

You can leave the talisman on your altar for as long as you feel is right. Some people like to leave them for a full moon cycle or even longer. When you feel complete, release the talisman back to the earth, ideally near the place where you harvested the herbs. This closes the circle and allows you to move forward in energetic freedom, into whatever comes next.

Chapter 10

Wild Oat

Common names: *wild oat, milky oat, oatstraw*

Latin name: *Avena spp. (spp. denotes species)*

Family: *Poaceae (grass family)*

Parts used: *mature seeds for cooking, immature flower heads and stems for herbal medicine*

This tall and slender plant really does live up to its name of "wild" as its seed heads sway back and forth in the breeze. Although wild oat has a reputation for blandness or even stodginess, it can help you reconnect with your own inner wildness. In modern parlance, the word *wild* is often taken to mean "unstable" or "crazy."

But wild oat reminds us of the inherent wildness of nature, of which we are a part. This herb can help you return to the wild state you enjoyed in childhood, before domestication and trauma taught you to be quiet, well-behaved, and predictable. It offers solace and deep replenishment to those trapped on the mainstream treadmill.

The Romans relied on this wild weed as a feed crop for their animals. It's thought that they brought it to the UK, where it flourished in the damp and cold climate of Scotland. Oat eventually replaced other crops as a mainstay for poor and working-class families, because it provided a very reliable staple when food was scarce. This humble wild member of the grass family now enjoys a place among esteemed Scottish traditions, and is grown in locations all around the world.

Habitat

Wild oat grows in many temperate regions around the globe, including Europe, North America, Asia, and parts of Australia. It thrives in areas with moderate temperatures and well-distributed rainfall.

The plant is adaptable and can grow in various soil types, from sandy and loamy soils to heavier clay. However, it prefers well-drained, fertile soils. It is commonly found in disturbed areas like fields, roadsides, and waste areas. It flourishes in cool, moist climates during its early growth stages, which is part of the reason it does so well in rainy Scotland.

Identification

Wild oat has a tall, slender stem that can grow as high as 60–150 cm (2–5'). The leaves are long, narrow, and flat, resembling typical grass leaves. They have a rough texture and can grow up to 45 cm (18") long. These leaves are arranged alternately along the stem, giving the plant a feathery appearance.

The flowers are small and green, and grow in clusters called panicles. These panicles can be 15–30 cm (6–12") long and are quite loose and open, allowing the small spikelets (flower clusters) to spread. Each spikelet contains two to three flowers with long, bristle-like structures called awns that help the seeds cling to fur or clothing, aiding in dispersal. A husk covers the elongated seeds, with a noticeable groove along one side. These hardy seeds are patient and can remain viable in the soil for several years, ready to sprout when conditions are right.

WILD OAT

Harvesting, Drying, and Storing

Unlike cultivated oats like wheat and barley, which are bred to grow and ripen uniformly, wild oat can be unpredictable in its ripening times. When the immature flower heads, commonly called fresh milky oat tops or simply milky oats, are squeezed, they yield a milky white fluid, and this is considered the optimal time for tincturing the plant. Identifying when they are at the milky stage (before full ripeness) takes a little practice, but I just pop the seeds (which I find immensely pleasurable) until I see the milky liquid emerge. As long as the majority of seeds are at this stage, even if a few aren't yet there or are a little more ripe than ideal, you can harvest them.

The dried stems, technically termed culms, are commonly known as oatstraw. They are rich in minerals and silica, and provide wonderful support for a depleted system. I recommend harvesting both the milky oats and the oatstraw at the same time, as it saves going back later. Cut the whole stalk 100–120 cm (3–4') from the top and stack them in the same direction to make processing easier. This gives you a combination of stalks, leaves, and seeds. Just remove any discolored leaves and place them in your compost bin.

Wild oat can be dried either passively or actively using a dehydrator set to 42°C (107°F) for twelve to fourteen hours. Remove the seeds from the stems and set them aside before drying, as these are best tinctured fresh. But be careful: oat can be a little mischievous! You may think your batch is completely dry, only to find it has gone moldy after a few weeks in storage. This only happened to me once, but it was a sad blow to lose my whole stock of the plant.

In his *Folk Flora*, Roy Vickery describes the traditional method of ensuring that the bundles of oat were dry before being stacked:

> They always used to say about oats, three Sundays after it was cut . . . Oats should have the church bells rung over them three times after they have been cut, i.e. must be left while the bells are tolled on three successive Sundays. Otherwise there will be sickness in the village.

Contraindications

Wild oat is generally safe and well tolerated, but of course you should avoid it if you have any known allergy to any type of oats.

There has been some confusion over whether oats are safe for those with celiac conditions because they contain a protein called avenin, which is a cousin of gluten. Nonetheless, research shows that those with these conditions can usually tolerate oats well, and that avenin does not create problems in the digestive tract. Despite this, I recommend buying oats certified as gluten-free if you are gluten-intolerant, as there has been known to be cross-contamination with other gluten-containing grains. And if you find that oats of any kind disagree with you, you should avoid working with them.

Four Sacred Medicines

Wild oat is one of the plants that cross the boundary between food and medicine. Here are some of the ways it can be used to treat ailments.

Physical Medicine

In physical medicine, wild oat is most commonly used to treat insomnia and skin conditions, and for cardiovascular support.

- *Insomnia:* Oatstraw and/or milky oats can be helpful for sleep-onset insomnia, when your head becomes filled with a cacophony of noise and thoughts the moment you lie down. It is also used to treat perimenopausal neurasthenia, a condition characterized by mental and/or physical fatigue accompanied by dizziness, dyspepsia, muscular aches or pains, tension headaches, inability to relax, irritability, and sleep disturbance.

- *Skin conditions*: Oatstraw infusions and porridge oats (the mature processed grain) can be used topically to reduce the itching, pain, and inflammation of chronic skin conditions like eczema and dermatitis.

- *Cardiovascular support*: When used as a food, oats are high in protein and soluble fiber, which research shows can support a healthy cardiovascular system, particularly when high blood pressure is an issue.[1]

Mental Medicine

If you are easily bored by people and situations, and constantly looking for distractions, wild oat can slow you down so you can enjoy where you are rather than thinking about where you would like to be. This reliable herb reminds you that there is wildness to be found in sitting still and allowing yourself to ripen slowly, rather than rushing on to the next thing.

Emotional Medicine

Wild oat is one of the best remedies for a depleted nervous system, especially when accompanied by chronic and ongoing stress of any kind, or when depression is born of exhaustion and anxiety. If you're thinking about so many things that you tire yourself out, wild oat can soothe and replenish you.

Spiritual Medicine

If you tend to look outside of yourself for answers and find it difficult to connect with your inner wisdom, the Spirit of Wild Oat can help you foster that connection. Stop looking for a guru who will change everything for you. Instead, seek out wild oat on a plant spirit journey to learn how to trust yourself, your insight, and your intuition. This can help you clarify your goals and your soul's purpose in life.

Working with Wild Oat

The next three practices give ways in which you can work with wild oat to connect with spirits associated with farming, community, and sharing.

Practice: Baking Bannocks

Bannocks are traditional Scottish flatbreads that are made from locally available grains like oat or barley and cooked on a griddle. In the past, people made and ate these breads together during festivals and gatherings to strengthen social bonds and enhance cultural continuity. They were used as both a food staple and as a means of invoking the blessings of the deities associated with the land and agriculture—something very important in times when the food supply was by no means assured.

Bannock recipes and preparation methods vary widely across Scotland. This tradition is diverse and adaptable, but the underlying principle is to use what you've got and share what you've made. You can share bannocks with friends or family, or give them as offerings to thank the spirits of the land.

For this recipe, you will need:

- 700ml (3 cups) oats

- ½ teaspoon baking soda

- ½ teaspoon salt

- 60ml (¼ cup) butter

● 250ml (1 cup) buttermilk or 250ml (1 cup) milk
mixed with 1 tablespoon lemon juice or white vinegar

Preheat the oven to 190°C (375°F). Grind the oats in a food processor until they resemble coarse flour. Save a small amount to dust your working surface when you knead the dough.

Combine the ground oats, baking soda, and salt in a large bowl. Cut the butter into small pieces and rub it into the dry mixture with your fingers until it resembles coarse crumbs. Make a well in the center of the mixture and pour in the buttermilk or buttermilk substitute. (If you are using a substitute, mix it ahead of time and let it sit for about five minutes until it curdles slightly.) Mix gently until the dough comes together, then turn it onto a surface that has been lightly dusted with the oat flour you saved. Knead the dough gently to combine the ingredients, then shape it into a round, flat disc about 12 mm (½") thick.

Place the dough on a greased baking sheet or a cast-iron skillet. Use a knife to score the top into wedges, cutting about halfway through the thickness of the dough. Bake in the preheated oven for twenty-five to thirty minutes, or until the bannock is golden brown and sounds hollow when tapped on the bottom.

Cool and serve with whatever fillings you like. You can add sweet or savory fillings, or enjoy it spread with butter.

Practice: Tasty Oatstraw Tea Blend

Try the following blend if you are feeling depleted after a stressful day, week, or month. If you are on thyroid medication, replace lemon balm with lemongrass in the same quantity.

- 2 parts oatstraw, dried and roughly chopped
- 1 part nettle leaf, dried and roughly chopped
- 1 part lemon balm, dried and roughly chopped

Place 1 heaped teaspoon of the combined herbs in a heat-resistant jug. Add 200ml (7 oz.) of freshly boiled water, cover, and infuse for fifteen to twenty minutes. Strain, pour into your favorite mug, and enjoy. You can sweeten the tea with honey if you prefer.

Practice: Oat Gratitude Ceremony

Ceremonies can serve many purposes. They mark rites of passage, celebrate milestones, and release and retrieve energy. The following is a ceremony of gratitude and offering to your plant spirit

WILD OAT

allies. The intimacy that comes from sharing food with another being is real and lasting, and has deep spiritual meaning in many cultures and religions.

In Celtic tradition, hospitality was a revered practice that was integral to social and spiritual life. Hosts were expected to provide generously for their guests, whether human or spirit. Reciprocity with the Otherworld involved offerings and rituals to honor and thank the spirits, ensuring their continued favor and protection.

To perform this ceremony, you will need:

- A bannock—either plain or with fillings, depending on your preference

- A beverage and two cups—any beverage you enjoy and hold in high regard (I like water, but make your own choice)

- Space for your bannock and drink offering on your plant spirit altar

- A quiet and peaceful place where you won't be disturbed

If you choose to perform this ceremony outside, you can craft an altar for this specific purpose, working with natural items around you. Whether working inside or out, cleanse yourself and open your space in your usual way, remembering to call in the spirit medicine of wild oat.

Sit comfortably and close your eyes. Take a few moments to breathe deeply and center yourself. Then open your eyes, take the bannock in your hands, and break it into three pieces. Place the first piece on your altar with this invocation:

> *I offer this bannock to the plant spirits, who protect,*
> *provide, illuminate, and guide. I offer this food in honor*
> *of you; please receive this gift given in love and gratitude.*

Pour the beverage into two cups and place one on the altar, saying:

> *I offer this drink and ask that you accept it. It is given freely*
> *and without obligation. It is given to honor the plant spirits.*

If you are outside, you can also pour some of the beverage directly onto the earth, saying:

WILD OAT

*I offer this drink to you, Mother Earth, keeper of the
cycle of life. Please accept this gift made in love and gratitude.*

Now it's your turn to eat. Pick up one of the remaining pieces of bannock and chew it mindfully, savoring the taste and texture. The earth has given generously so you can eat and you should respect this. You can also drink your beverage. You'll most likely need it by this time, as oats and bannocks, while tasty, are notoriously dry!

When you have finished your meal, if you are outside, place your offerings on the ground so they can return to the earth. Consuming offerings made to the spirits was seen by traditional peoples as a violation of an important reciprocal relationship that could lead to potential misfortune—a breaking of sacred trust. Once food is gifted to the spirits, it no longer belongs to you. So gift it back to the earth after the conclusion of your ceremony.

Close your sacred space by thanking the plant spirits that were present, saying:

This space is now closed, but my gratitude continues to flow.

PLANT SPIRIT HERBALISM

Part IV

PLANT SPIRIT ALLIES FOR SUMMER

The beginning of summer is a precious time when leaves are a shimmering, otherworldly green, like a ripe Granny Smith apple. The plants that weathered the storms of spring are growing to maturity. Flower buds swell and open; leaves unfurl and turn their faces to greet the sun. The roots that burrowed deep in winter fulfill their promise in these months of light.

During this potent time, we become more sensitive to the higher energies present in the natural world. Sometimes we need to "turn down the volume" and protect our boundaries and energetic space. As the path of the sun rises higher in the sky, our bodies adapt by increasing blood flow to the skin to dissipate the extra heat. We sweat more frequently as our bodies work to maintain a constant temperature. Just like the newly planted herbs in our gardens, we are thirstier and need to be "watered" each day.

During the sun-drenched days of summer, our bodies put forth extra effort. Our hearts, our nerves, our skin, and all our organs feel the heat. We are more susceptible to skin conditions. Days are long and nights are short, so sleep patterns suffer. Outdoor adventures cause an increase in minor injuries—scrapes from tree-climbing or sprains from hiking. Although summer is associated with vacations and fun, it can also be a time of high stress as we attempt to cram ever more activities into our schedules and keep children entertained.

Herbal allies for this season support our hardworking bodies and help us manage these challenges. They embody the energies of the sun and remind us to relax and enjoy the ride. They tell us to take time to swing in a hammock or lie on a riverbank instead of rushing on to the next adventure. These cooling, soothing herbs relax us, diffuse heat, and offer practical first aid.

Chapter 11

Hawthorn

Common names: *hawthorn, bread and butter, bread and cheese*
Latin name: *Crataegus spp.*
Family: *Rosaceae*
Parts used: *flower and leaf in spring and summer, berry in autumn*

I live in the foothills of the Cairngorm Mountains in Scotland, where hedgerows and stone walls are still important boundary markers, not yet completely overtaken by metal fencing. Hawthorn is one of those important hedgerow trees whose thorns provide an excellent deterrent to any animals seeking to escape their fields, while providing a wonderful haven for wildlife—indeed, some three hundred species of insects call this plant home.

There's an old Scottish folk saying that warns: "Ne'er cast a clout till May is oot." Which means that you should wait until hawthorn is in bloom until you change from your thick, heavy winter clothes to your lighter summer garb. Where I live, that's mid-May, and it seems like an eternity when I hear of trees blooming weeks before in southern regions!

The early spring leaves of hawthorn were once eaten as a snack by children on their way to school, and one of its common names is bread and butter, or bread and cheese. The origin of these names is unclear, but folk evidence points to several possible explanations. One theory is that hawthorn leaves were used as a kind of rennet substitute to make cheese and other fermented foods like bread, and were named this way to seem more appealing when food was scarce. Another explanation is that the appetizing-looking red hawthorn berries were rather bland—like bread and butter. Whatever the origins, the young leaves make a tasty snack with a nutty, almost lemony taste. As with most edible leaves, it is best to get them when they are young and tender.

Hawthorn is a plant of paradox. It is associated with protection and healing if treated with proper respect, but is linked to bad luck if used incorrectly or disrespected. A London-based folklore group once did a study on references to "unlucky" plants found in traditional sources, and 23.4 percent of their findings were concerned with hawthorn![1] But there are just as many accounts of hawthorn being sacred and protective.

Lone hawthorns are particularly auspicious, and the space around them is believed to be a portal to the unseen realms. Whole roads and underground sewer systems have been rerouted to avoid damaging lone hawthorn trees.

Habitat

This plant is native to northern temperate zones, including Western Europe and the UK, but it is found around the globe, from the coasts of North America to parts of Australia and New Zealand. It is commonly found growing in hedgerows, woodland, and scrub. It will grow in most soils, but flowers and fruits best in full sun.

Identification

Mature hawthorn trees can reach a height of 15 m (50') and are characterized by their dense, thorny branches, but they can also grow as small trees with a single stem. Their knotted and fissured bark is brown-gray. The twigs are slender and brown, and covered in thorns. Look out for the deeply lobed leaves, spiny twigs, and haws (berries) of this plant. Spines, which emerge from the same point as the buds, identify hawthorn in winter. This distinguishes it from blackthorn (*Prunus spinosa*), which has no spines. Unlike hawthorn, blackthorn flowers before it produces leaves.

Harvesting, Drying, and Storing

Harvest hawthorn flowers when they still have pink ends on the pollen, as this is when they are at their most medicinal. Flowering can start as early as mid-April or as late as the end of May in some more northern areas. The seeds of the berries contain cyanogenic glycosides (called amygdalin), a potentially toxic chemical, so avoid ingesting the seeds of the fresh berry. Fortunately, this is easy to do, because the seeds are quite large.

Hawthorn flowers and berries grow on multiple little stalks that sprout from the branch. Using secateurs, snip these and place them facing down in your basket to allow any insects to escape. You can also harvest the leaves, as they are medicinal as well.

It is best not to wash hawthorn flowers, as they will turn to mush and you will lose some of the medicinal pollen. You can wash the berries, however. The drying or preparation process will be sufficient to remove anything unwanted.

Place the berries in a bowl of fresh, cold water and discard any that are very discolored. Remove the berries from the stalk before drying them or processing them into a syrup or fresh tincture.

Dry the flower heads whole, either on or off the stalk. If they are still on the stalk, remove them after you have dried them. Aim for dry, papery, crisp, but still creamy-colored flowers. You can dry passively or using a dehydrator set to 42°C (107°F) for twelve hours or overnight.

Contraindications

Hawthorn has no known contraindications. However, when you are ingesting the physical medicine of hawthorn, try to avoid large doses or use it in a blend if constipation is an issue. Hawthorn berries are sour and astringent, and may make constipation worse. If you are taking medications for your heart, exercise caution. I encourage you to work with an herbalist or naturopath.

Four Sacred Medicines

All species of hawthorn are medicinal and can be found worldwide. It has a broad range of uses across all four healing modalities.

Physical Medicine

You can work with hawthorn leaves, berries, and flowers. I like to combine all three when making a tincture or infusion.

- *Cardiovascular support*: Taking this herb regularly can help keep blood vessels clear of atheroma, the plaque that builds up in arteries and leads to heart disease. It also supports the heart muscle and lowers blood pressure by making it easier for blood to flow. I work with hawthorn for conditions like angina, congestive heart failure, and high and low blood pressure, as it helps the body find balance without forcing change.

- *Nervous system*: Hawthorn gently prompts the vagus nerve to swing into action, triggering what's called the parasympathetic response—a natural relaxation switch for the body. It helps you unwind and aids digestion—both of which can be very good things in the frenetic days of summer.

- *Joint health*: If lawn-mowing and other summertime chores have set your joints aching, hawthorn can reduce inflammation in the connective tissues and ease the symptoms of arthritis, gout, and tendonitis.

Mental Medicine

I've lost count of the number of times I've been walking along, stuck in my own head, and literally gotten tangled in the hawthorn bushes that line the path. Hawthorn helps me to "be here now," pulling me out of ruminative thoughts and back into the present moment.

Emotional Medicine

Hawthorn is invaluable for healing long-held hurt and trauma, especially if you have processed what happened in your mind, but your body has yet to catch up. It is also a key ally in times of grief. It won't magically remove the pain, but it can provide powerful support, a listening ear, and some solace when you see no clear way forward.

Spiritual Medicine

The spirit medicine of hawthorn helps you accept yourself exactly as you are and counsels you to allow love into your heart. It offers protection against psychic intrusions and unwanted energies.

Like vigilant sentinels, its spiny thorns stand as guardians of boundaries. In plant spirit journeys, hawthorn can show up to help you realize when you are taking on too much. It reminds you that setting limits is essential for your well-being. Just as its thorns protect hawthorn blossoms, they encourage you to protect your inner self from intrusions and teach that discomfort and challenges are stepping stones to growth.

Hawthorn flowers produce an organic compound called trimethylamine (TMA) that has a curious odor—one that also occurs when humans have sex and when animals decompose! This serves as a reminder of this plant's association with sacred sexuality, fertility, and death, both in the metaphorical sense— the small endings and beginnings we all experience as we move through life—and the literal sense—the big "ending" that comes to us all.

Working with Hawthorn

These three practices call on the Spirit of Hawthorn to help you reach down into the hidden parts of your emotional world and make big changes.

Practice: Hawberry Ketchup

You have to wait until autumn to try this recipe. But if you really can't wait, you can purchase dried hawthorn berries. Soften the dried berries first by simmering them in water for approximately fifteen to twenty minutes.

To make this ketchup, you will need:

- 500g (1 lb.) fresh hawthorn berries
- 350ml (1½ cups) water
- 350ml (1½ cups) apple cider vinegar
- 150g (5 oz.) soft brown sugar
- A pinch of salt and pepper
- ¼ teaspoon ground ginger (optional)
- ¼ teaspoon ground cinnamon (optional)

Start by removing any shriveled, damaged, or moldy berries. Rinse and drain the remaining berries and place them in a saucepan with water and the apple cider vinegar. Simmer for thirty minutes, or until the skins split and the flesh is softened.

Now comes the laborious part. Place the softened berries in a sieve, and scrape and push as much fruit flesh through as possible. The longer you spend doing this, the better your final product will be, trust me!

Return the fruit pulp to the pan and add the remaining ingredients. Simmer gently, stirring regularly until the mixture reaches your preferred thickness (five to fifteen minutes usually does it). Note that the mixture will thicken more as it cools. Pour the ketchup into a sterile jar and refrigerate it once it has cooled.

Use this heart-healthy sauce anytime you need a delicious condiment!

Practice: Hawthorn Flower Essence

Flower essences are subtle herbal medicines that are used in a form so dilute and in quantities so small that they can reach down into the hidden parts of your emotional world and help you make big changes. They access areas that are off-limits to the bigger, bolder herbal tinctures and teas.

Less is definitely more with flower essences. In a culture that defines success by how much you accumulate and how much you consume, it can be tempting to take more than the recommended few drops of these essences. But if you do, you will simply be wasting your medicine and not increasing its healing potential.

To make your own hawthorn flower essence, you will need:

- Hawthorn flowers

- A simple, small glass bowl (avoid metal, plastic, and crystal)

- Spring water or distilled water

- Good-quality brandy (unflavored) or food-grade glycerine (if you want to avoid alcohol)

- 2 glass storage bottles, 50–100ml (2–4 oz.)

- Several glass treatment bottles, 20–50ml (½–2 oz.)

This essence should be prepared in either sunlight or moonlight, depending on the type of essence you're making.

Begin by gathering the hawthorn flowers on a sunny day, or on or near a Full Moon, as appropriate. If you are working with fresh flowers, gather them at the peak of flowering. Avoid touching them directly at any point during harvesting or preparation. I like to use a large dock leaf and scissors to hold and snip the flowers into my basket. Then I use chopsticks to transfer them onto the water's surface. If you are working with dried flowers, I recommend purifying them by smoke cleansing first.

Fill the glass bowl almost to the top with spring or distilled water. Float the flowers on the water's surface, again using a leaf or chopsticks to avoid touching them. The surface of the water should be well covered, but the blossoms should not overlap. Leave them to soak in the sunlight or moonlight for three to four hours, until they start to fade and the water is full of joyful little bubbles.

Fill a storage bottle half full with brandy or glycerine, then strain the water in the bowl into the bottle. This is your mother essence. It will last a lifetime if made with brandy, and up to five years if made with glycerine. You can use the leftover water and used flowers to make more mother essence, or give it to the earth as an offering.

The next step is to prepare your flower essence for consumption. Fill a second storage bottle half full with brandy or glycerine and add spring water to almost fill the bottle. Then add five drops of your mother essence, cap tightly, and shake vigorously. Below, I call this your "stock bottle." You can make more of these stock bottles if you need them. Just follow the steps above.

Finally, create the treatment bottles from which you will actually consume the medicine in drop form. Fill one of the smaller bottles with a mixture of 1 part glycerine or brandy and 3 parts spring water. Then add four to five drops from your stock bottle and cap it tightly. Shake the bottle well and label it. You can make more of these bottles as required. Just follow the steps above.

When you feel the need for support from the spirit of Hawthorn, place three to five drops of the mixture in the treatment bottle under your tongue or dilute them in water and drink. You can do this three or more times daily. But remember, using more drops per dose will not give you a better result. It will just waste your essence. Flower essences can also be added to healing creams, tinctures, teas, or lotions.

Practice: Hawthorn Ceremony—Be Here Now

If the swirl of summer activities has fried your nerves and set your head spinning, hawthorn can bring you into the present moment and help you to "be here now." In this ceremony, you call on the Spirit of Hawthorn to help you gently release mental overload and appreciate what *is*.

To perform this ceremony, all you need is a quiet and comfortable space to sit or lie down, a hawthorn tree or photograph

HAWTHORN   171

or drawing of one, and your journal and pen to record your experience.

Find a comfortable spot where you can sit near a hawthorn tree or with a photograph or drawing of one. Open your sacred space using words like: "I call upon the Spirit of Hawthorn," or "I ask hawthorn to be present during this ceremony." State your intention to come into the present moment and ask for hawthorn's assistance.

Sit in this space, gently paying attention to whatever comes from the spirit of the plant. You may feel physical sensations in your body. You may hear messages or sense emotions. Or you may experience something else entirely. Simply stay open to whatever arises within; observe it without judgment and from a place of compassion.

If old memories surface, give them thanks for being there. If irritations or impulses arise, bring in compassion. Know that hawthorn is offering these impressions as a form of gentle cleansing, showing you what you need to release in order to be fully present.

When you feel complete, open your eyes and give heartfelt thanks to the plant spirit. Be as detailed as possible, and avoid offering just a cursory "Thank you." Close your space and record your experience in your journal.

Chapter 12

Yarrow

Common names: *yarrow, soldier's woundwort*
Latin name: *Achillea millefolium*
Family: *Asteraceae (daisy)*
Parts used: *young leaves and flower heads*

Yarrow has such delicate white flowers and graceful leaves that you might not notice it at first glance among the showier herbs amid which it grows. Do not let appearances fool you, however. This herb is a powerhouse. If I were stuck on a desert island and had to choose one herb to have with me, I might choose this one!

The day I met yarrow was like so many others during the school holidays, which means I was outside on an adventure with my children. We had ventured out to a local nature reserve and had a vast stretch of loch and forests to explore. We had to navigate over many stiles—fences with built-in ladders—to get down to the water's edge and roam freely. One particular stile had sharp and unforgiving barbed wire on top. In my distracted state trying to wrangle children and picnics across the landscape, I caught my leg on this vicious wire and gave myself a deep wound that would not stop bleeding.

Luckily for me, the area where we were hiking had the type of soil that yarrow loves—thin, rough, and sandy. No rich and manicured gardens for this herb! Although I hadn't worked with yarrow before, I knew its key action was to stop bleeding and I was willing to try anything at that point. So I reached down, plucked a young leaf, put it in my mouth to mash it up, and placed it on the wound. This is called a "spit poultice," and it's ideal if you're in a bind and need medicine fast. Just don't make them for others; to reduce the risk of infection, get them to make their own.

When I applied the yarrow, three things happened. The bleeding stopped almost instantly; the wound began to tingle with the promise of healing and disinfection; and my mouth was filled with an intense bitter taste that left me unable to speak for several minutes. It was the type of bitterness that might make a young child cry.

My wound healed quickly and without scarring or infection, proving how powerful yarrow can be. And the intensely bitter taste and my body's reaction to it showed me that yarrow stimulates digestion and brings us back into the present moment via a reflex reaction of the nervous system. Yarrow came to my rescue that day, much as a knight in shining armor might rescue a damsel in distress. Now, yarrow has become one of my closest herbal allies.

Historically, yarrow was used on battlefields to staunch bleeding and clean wounds. Thus its name *Achillea millefolium*—after the Greek hero and warrior Achilles—is apt. Yarrow indeed heals all physical, mental, emotional, and spiritual wounds.

In Scotland, there are many folktales and incantations associated with yarrow. One of my favorites, which was recited aloud by herbalists as they gathered the plant, paints a vivid picture of its action.[1] I encourage you to read this out loud and sit with the power of the words.

> *I will pluck the yarrow fair,*
> *The more brave shall be my hand,*

YARROW

The more warm shall be my lips,

That more swift shall be my foot;

May I be an island at sea,

May I be a rock on land,

That I can afflict any man,

No man can afflict me.

Powerful words for such an unassuming plant. It speaks to the medicine of protection and courage, moving blood and supporting circulation. Yarrow is all of these things and more.

Yarrow was also used in divination rites in Scotland by those who wanted to determine their future lovers. Young girls plucked it on Beltaine morning while reciting a rhyme and placed it under their pillows that evening. Folk legend has it that their lovers would be revealed to them in their dreams, or by how a certain person acted in the days that followed.

Habitat

Due to its hardy nature, yarrow thrives in various habitats. It is commonly seen in meadows, fields, roadsides, disturbed areas, and open grasslands. It can adapt to different soil types, but prefers well-drained soils.

Identification

Yarrow has feathery, fern-like leaves that produce small white or pink flower clusters. Its leaves alternate and are deeply dissected down to a central rib. They are arranged along the stem in a spiral pattern, usually about 7–10 cm (3–4") long.

Yarrow flowers grow in flat-topped clusters called umbels. These clusters consist of numerous small, individual flowers with a diameter of 6–12 mm (¼–½"). They bloom from late spring to early fall, depending on the region. You will most likely see the characteristic flower clusters during this period.

Yarrow grows 30–90 cm (1–3') tall, but I have seen it grow to more than 120 cm (4') in rich soil. The reddish or greenish stems are erect, sturdy, and slightly hairy. Due to its spreading rhizomes, the plant often forms dense clumps.

Yarrow has a distinctive, somewhat spicy or medicinal scent when the leaves or flowers are crushed. The aroma can help confirm identification.

Harvesting, Drying, and Storing

To harvest yarrow leaves, you can snip them off at the base if the flowers haven't started growing. Or you can use the smaller leaves near the top of the plant if it is in flower. To harvest the blossoms, snip the whole flower head and some stalk just below the smaller leaves. If possible, leave your harvest outside for a few hours to ensure that any tiny critters have a chance to escape.

Yarrow stalks should break cleanly when dry; there should be no bending when you try to fold them. The leaves should crumble when rubbed through your fingers. You can dry yarrow passively or actively with a dehydrator set to 42°C (107°F) for twelve hours.

Once dried, remove the leaves and flower heads from the stalks and store them in an airtight container. You can discard the stalks or, if you want to work with yarrow-stalk divination, you can keep them until you have enough.

Contraindications

Avoid this plant during pregnancy or if you have any known allergy to the *Compositae* (daisy) family.

Four Sacred Medicines

We've already seen how yarrow can be used to treat wounds, but it has many other properties as well, including the ability to heal mental, emotional, and spiritual trauma.

Physical Medicine

Yarrow focuses on the digestive tract, circulation, skin, and female reproductive organs, as well as on healing wounds.

- *Digestive system*: As a bitter herb high in volatile oils, yarrow is effective for treating loss of appetite, heartburn, bloating, painful spasms, and gas in the lower and upper intestinal tracts. It indirectly stimulates the liver by improving blood flow and increasing bile production. A fresh infusion of the herb (combining leaf and flower) can ease digestive discomfort. For those who don't like the taste of yarrow, combine it with pleasant-tasting herbs like peppermint (*Mentha piperita* spp.) or lemon balm (*Melissa officinalis*).

- *Circulation*: Yarrow contains compounds that promote the dilation of blood vessels, causing them to relax and widen, thus improving blood flow. This may help with issues related to poor circulation, like cold hands and feet. It also reduces strain on the heart, as blood flows more easily through the vessels.

- *Blood clots*: Yarrow contains bioactive compounds that have anticoagulant properties that can prevent blood clots—vascular obstructions that can potentially lead to serious conditions like deep vein thrombosis or stroke.

- *Skin conditions*: You can apply fresh or dried yarrow leaves topically as a poultice to wounds to stop bleeding, prevent infection, and promote healing. I carry some dried and powdered yarrow leaf with me whenever I am out and about to use for first aid. I sprinkle it liberally and directly onto the wound.

- *Internal bleeding*: The dried leaf and flower of yarrow can be taken internally to address bleeding hemorrhoids and hemoptysis (blood coughed up from the respiratory tract).

- *Reproductive system*: Used in a sitz bath or full bath, yarrow flower and leaf can provide relief from lower pelvic pain and cramping. They can also help ease heavy, painful menstrual flow and bring on periods that have stopped (amenorrhea). This seemingly opposite action is true for many herbs. Herbs act to balance; in this case, yarrow balances blood flow. As the famous herbalist Maud Grieve wrote: "It seems to act either way."

Mental Medicine

If you are filled with anger at seemingly innocuous events, yarrow can connect you with the root of this rage, shining a light on subconscious and hidden trauma. If you struggle to undertake a task or have a difficult conversation, holding yarrow and nettle in your hand can help you summon up courage and determination. I have used this technique countless times, with wonderful results.

Emotional Medicine

This herb supports transitions of any kind. It gives you courage and energy to move through an experience and come out the other side. As a balancer, it regulates mood swings during hormonal shifts, like those experienced during perimenopause and menopause.

Yarrow is also an herb for lovers, as we saw in the Beltaine tradition described above. Another folk legend encouraged young women to cut yarrow flowers before sunrise, put them under their pillows, and hope to dream of their sweethearts. If a young man faced a woman in the dream, they would marry. But if he faced away from her, they were not destined to wed. Today, this divination tool can be used regardless of your age, gender, or sexual orientation.

Spiritual Medicine

Yarrow is powerful medicine. This plant spirit ally can give you the courage to face your deepest fears and even overcome your own "Achilles heel," providing energetic protection while you carry out sacred work. It's the perfect bodyguard to carry with you in crowded or hectic places, or when you have to attend a stressful event.

Working with yarrow can also help develop your psychic ability—called "second sight" in Scotland. In Gaelic, the term for second sight is *da-shealladh,* meaning "two worlds," pointing to the existence of a realm beyond what most can ordinarily see.

Working with Yarrow

These two practices can help you draw on the healing powers of this versatile plant.

Practice: Yarrow First Aid Powder

As you have already learned, yarrow is excellent for stopping bleeding and disinfecting wounds. As summer takes you outside on more adventures, powdered yarrow is a good thing to carry with you. It's simple to make, but incredibly effective. The young leaves are high in the tannins that stop bleeding, and the flowers contain more of the phenolic compounds and volatile oils that give this herb its anti-inflammatory and antimicrobial action.

Collect the young leaves in spring and dry them whole. When the plant flowers, collect the flowering tops and dry them whole as well. Then strip the dried leaves off the main stem and pull the dried flower heads off the stalks. The stalks and stems are difficult to grind and powder, and can make your final product a little coarse.

Grind the leaves and flower heads in a grinder or with a mortar and pestle until finely powdered and store in a small, dark glass jar. Sprinkle the powder on cuts and scrapes. For larger wounds, of course, I always recommend seeking medical attention.

Practice: Yarrow Medicine Pouch

We have all had times when we needed to step up and enter a space that we may not have felt equipped to handle. And we've all had times when we turned ourselves inside out and tied ourselves in knots because we really wanted to do something but couldn't bring ourselves to do it.

I work closely with yarrow during times like these, especially when I find myself procrastinating, doing anything but undertaking what I so desperately want to do. Yarrow is a plant of the battlefield. It can help you find your courage! And medicine pouches are one of my favorite ways to connect with this aspect of herbal medicine. Carrying herbs with you in a medicine pouch is an easy and effective way to harness a plant spirit's medicine and keep it close at hand. They act as tangible links and remind you that you have an ally by your side.

To make this medicine pouch, you will need:

- A small handful of dried yarrow

- A clean and empty bowl

- A small square of cloth

- A piece of string to tie the cloth up into a small pouch

Cleanse yourself and open your space in your usual way, being sure to call on the Spirit of Yarrow. Take some gentle breaths and sink into the stillness that comes with ritual preparation.

When you feel ready, pick up the dried yarrow, close your eyes, and feel the textures of the herb in your hand. Really connect with the sensations. Does the herb feel soft? Hard? Spiky? Then raise it to your nose and appreciate its fragrance. Take your time. You may feel your body start to respond to the volatile oils as they hit the olfactory nerves in your nose.

Slowly crumble the yarrow into smaller pieces and drop them into the clean bowl. As you do this, chant the following words over and over until you have finished crumbling the herbs:

Yarrow connects me to my courage.

Yarrow stands by my side. Yarrow is my ally.

Place the crumbled herb in the center of the piece of fabric and gather the four corners together. Then tie the pouch tightly with string, making sure that you knot it well so that it doesn't come undone.

Tuck this courage-making medicine pouch into your pocket or clothing. If you feel yourself avoiding a task you want to do, or hesitating to have a conversation you need to have, reach in and grasp the pouch, knowing that this powerful ally is by your side and that your courage is with you as well.

Chapter 13

Lemon Balm

Common names: *lemon balm, bee balm, balm*
Latin name: *Melissa officinalis*
Family: *Lamiaceae*
Parts used: *aerial parts, leaf and stem*

Lemon balm thrives where other plants may struggle, pushing up through dry, dusty earth. This herb is forgiving and doesn't ask that you be a spectacular, seasoned gardener. Instead, it is tenacious and self-sufficient. This intrepid member of the mint family makes its way happily around your garden with little assistance from you.

Lemon balm has a peculiar effect on me, regardless of my mood. If I chew on small pieces or spend some time in its company, I smile and have the overwhelming urge to move my body and dance. A joyful, uplifting, almost euphoric feeling washes over me, after which I feel calm, reset, and refreshed, regardless of how I was feeling before. Unflinching, holding space, lighting the way, helping me carry my burden—I simply couldn't imagine life without lemon balm!

There is a rich medical and folkloric history attached to this herb. Paracelsus (1493–1541) stated that lemon balm would "completely revivify a man" and should be used for "all complaints supposed to proceed from a disordered state of the nervous system." It was said to possess the ability to rejuvenate anyone who partook of it—high praise indeed for an herb! The first word of this plant's Latin name, *Melissa*, is Greek for "bee," and bees love this herb when it's in flower. As Pliny the Elder wrote,

> Bees are delighted with this herbe above all others . . . when they are straid away, they do finde their way home againe by it . . . It is of so great virtue that though it be but tied to his sword that hath given the wound it stauncheth the blood.

The second word of its name, *officinalis*, comes from the name for the building where mediaeval monks prepared their medicines. It is interesting to note that, when Linnaeus first developed the nomenclature that we still use to classify plants today, he assigned the term *officinalis* to herbs with documented uses. He gave this name to dozens of different herbs, thus tagging them as having proven medicinal properties.

Habitat

Native to the south of Europe, this herb was then introduced into the UK and mainland America. If you find lemon balm growing in the wild, it is likely an escapee from a garden. Escaped plants are typically found in habitats like vacant lots, roadsides, banks of ponds, floodplains along drainage canals, and waste areas. They prefer locations with a history of human disturbance, as well as sites that are not too sunny or damp. They like a happy balance of light and moisture. That said, I've seen lemon balm growing in several places that don't meet these requirements. This plant is both gentle and tenacious.

Identification

This bushy, perennial herb typically stands 30–90 cm (1–3') tall. The stems are light green with four sides, which is typical of the mint family. They can be smooth or slightly hairy. The oval-shaped leaves grow in opposing pairs along the stem, and get smaller as you move up the stem. The tips of the leaves are rounded and the bottom part is wider, forming a wedge shape with serrated edges. Crushing the leaves gives off a lovely lemony aroma that varies in strength depending on the cultivar and sun exposure.

Bunches of two to ten small white flowers grow from the spots where the upper leaves meet the stem, held up by short stems that are 1–5 mm (⅛–¼") long.

Harvesting, Drying, and Storing

In spring and early summer, harvest the whole stalks with the leaf attached. Later in the season, when stalks are longer and more twig-like, drying becomes more difficult. At this stage, I recommend that you leave the stalks and harvest only the leaf.

You can dry lemon balm passively or actively with a dehydrator set to 42°C (107°F) for nine to twelve hours or overnight.

Contraindications

Avoid high doses if you are in active treatment for hypothyroidism.

Four Sacred Medicines

Lemon balm is a simple herb that is active across all four healing modalities.

Physical Medicine

This herb's physical properties cover a number of common ailments, ranging from insomnia to infection control.

- *Insomnia*: Lemon balm is helpful for insomnia, especially when overthinking or mood disorders make it difficult to get to sleep and stay there.

- *Digestive system*: This plant can ease indigestion, cramping, flatulence, bloating, and burping, especially when these symptoms worsen when stress is present. The bitter action helps to support the liver and gallbladder, thereby enhancing the digestion and absorption of food.

- *Colic*: Lemon balm is a wonderful remedy for colic in babies and young children. Combine it in a tea with fennel and chamomile to treat children, or bathe infants in a strong infusion if they are still exclusively breast- or bottle-fed.

- *Nervous system*: This is a great example of an herb that provides balance. It can help to relax and calm when tension, irritability, and anxiety are present. It uplifts and provides support for forward movement in instances of low mood and depression. I love to combine this plant with St. John's Wort to support seasonal mood changes like seasonal affective disorder.

- *Reproductive system*: The relaxing action of lemon balm can help reduce the pain and spasms of menstruation, and help with mood changes common in PMS and perimenopause.

- *Infection*: I often combine this herb with yarrow and elderberries in a hot infusion to treat fevers due to infections like the common cold. Its astringent properties can also reduce mucus buildup in the lungs during an infection.

- *Antimicrobial*: Lemon balm can be used both topically and internally as an antiviral and antimicrobial, helping the body fight off infections. Make a strong infusion for cold sores and apply it directly to the sore. Remember to use a clean cotton swab each time to avoid introducing viral material into the infusion. The earlier you start treatment, the better the results will be with cold sores. Stored in the refrigerator, this infusion will last up to forty-eight hours.

- *Blood pressure support*: Combined with linden blossom, lemon balm is excellent for lowering blood pressure and relieving the physical effects of anxiety, like palpitations and racing heartbeat.

Mental Medicine

Lemon balm's cool, collected nature can slow down your thoughts. Rather than trying to think your way out of a problem, let lemon balm help you be still, be present, and listen to what is unfolding. This enables you to see things from a slightly different perspective—just enough so that you can find a clear way through.

Emotional Medicine

If your mood is low and you're struggling to find a reason to get up and get moving, lemon balm can provide the little spark you need to get going. It brings you a bit of joy when it's in short supply. This herb won't magically make you feel better, but it will provide some reassuring assistance as you move forward.

Spiritual Medicine

Lemon balm is a protective herb that surrounds you with a comforting green mantle that repels unwanted energies and keeps your energetic boundaries safe. The many connections of this plant to the sacred bee and to goddesses indicate its associations with feminine mysteries. Connecting with it can thus help you soften your perspective and rest before taking action, so that you can see more clearly and from a soul-led place.

Lemon balm encourages you to stay a while in the dark, so that your movement into the light aligns with your divine spirit. Most important, it gladdens the heart and helps you unlock your intuition and insight. It is the perfect herb to use in spirit journeys, meditation, and dream work.

Working with Lemon Balm

These two practices let you unlock the unique powers of lemon balm and bring its calming magic into your life.

Practice: Aromatic Lemon Balm Syrup

This simple recipe yields a delicious syrup you can use to flavor a refreshing drink, or take alone as a calming tonic.

To make this syrup, you will need:

- Fresh lemon balm tops—enough to fill a canning jar

- A sterilized glass canning jar with lid

- Vegetable glycerin

- Water

- A pan of boiling water (or a canner if you have one)

Roughly chop the lemon balm and fill the canning jar with the chopped herb. Make sure the jar is completely full by pressing the herbs down lightly and adding more if necessary.

Make a solution of 70 percent glycerin and 30 percent water and pour it into the jar until the herbs are completely covered. Cap the jar and seal it tightly to prevent the aromatic oils from escaping. Place the sealed canning jar into a pan of boiling water or canner and let it simmer for fifteen to twenty minutes, then remove. When the jar is cool to the touch, open it and strain out the herbs.

The fragrance released during this process is incredible. The sweet flavor of the glycerine disguises the slightly bitter taste of the lemon balm. This makes an excellent syrup to add to sparkling mineral water for a refreshing drink. Or take it directly off a spoon as a tasty medicine—a rare thing in the herb world.

Practice: Lemon Balm Bath Ritual

You can use herbs topically in many ways, but adding them to your bathwater is the easiest and most fun. As an herbalist, I often recommend that clients work with a certain herb topically to help soothe skin conditions or as added support for the nervous system or hormone balancing. If full-body bathing is not possible for you, you can use a large tub and just soak your hands or feet.

Hot water has its own benefits, the alchemy of fire and water combining into a pleasurable blend of heat and steam. When I get into a bath or shower, I always start by giving thanks to the spirits of water and fire for letting me enjoy the luxury of hot water. This turns an everyday action into a sacred act.

Hot water boosts circulation to your arms and legs and opens your pores. This makes it easier for an herb's active properties to be absorbed through the skin. It also helps relax your muscles and encourages them to give up tension and tightness for a short while. When you take a hot bath, you don't need to "hold" anything. You can put down your burdens for a little while. When you add herbs to the mix, the health benefits increase. You can use herbs every time you bathe, or when you need them to soothe a skin irritation. Or you can incorporate herbal baths into a regular weekly or monthly ritual. The choice is yours.

This lemon balm bath ritual gives you an opportunity to pause during the energetic outward-directed season of summer. It provides a chance to reflect on your progress and assess what you can alter and readjust to ensure that the goals you set in the darkness of early spring still align with your inner wisdom. Lemon balm can help bring success to whatever aspect of your life you are addressing. All you need for this simple ritual is a large handful of roughly chopped fresh lemon balm leaves and stems (or 50g (1.8 oz.) of the dried herb), and 500ml (1 pint) of freshly boiled water.

Begin by adding the chopped herb to the freshly boiled water. Cover and leave the mixture to infuse for fifteen minutes. Covering the infusion keeps the volatile oils—the ingredient in the herb that gives it its aroma and medicine—from escaping.

While the herb is infusing, set your sacred bath space. Clean the tub thoroughly before filling it with water. I like to make sure that the rest of the bathroom is tidy as well, removing any toys, laundry, or clutter. Sometimes I light candles or put wildflowers in a vase. I set the intention that this time is for *me*. If other people or pets want to get involved, I put up a firm boundary. This is my time to rest and rejuvenate. You cannot pour from an empty cup and, if you have kids, showing them that your needs matter also shows them the importance of meeting their own needs.

Fill the tub with water, making sure the temperature feels exactly right for you in that moment. When you are ready, retrieve the infusion you made and strain it. You can skip this step if you like plant parts floating in your bathwater. Add the infusion directly to your bath, inhaling the pleasantly fresh, lemony fragrance.

When you first get into the tub, take a moment to thank the spirits of water and fire. Spend some time enjoying the aroma, knowing that your physical body is benefiting from this wonderful herb. Relax into the medicine of lemon balm. Close your eyes and give thanks for the nourishment it provides your nervous system and muscles. Then reflect on how you are spending the summer season. Are you living the fullness of what you dreamed into being in the dark of winter? Or do you need to adjust your course?

Let the hot water and lemon balm hold you, and when you have completed your reflections, let it all go. Just rest in silence. In this quiet space, let your soul commune with your plant allies to manifest the intention of your ceremony. Make any adjustments to your course that are necessary in order to keep you aligned with your soul journey. Take your time; you don't need to be *doing* anything. Just *be*. You may receive flashes of insight. You may feel sensations in your body. You may get a sense of a change you need to make. Or you may experience something else entirely. Stay open to whatever comes up.

LEMON BALM

When you feel ready, give thanks to the Spirit of Lemon Balm and to the elements that supported this transformative experience. Close your space by saying:

This space is now closed, but blessings continue to flow.

Drain the bath and douse any candles you lit, knowing that whatever has been released from you during this bath ritual will be transmuted into loving fertilizer for the earth.

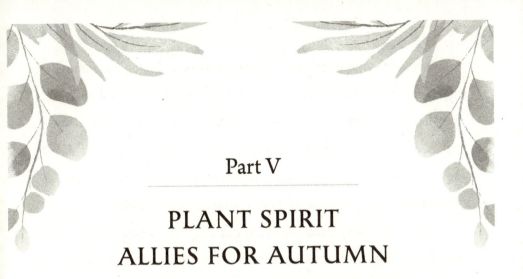

Part V

PLANT SPIRIT ALLIES FOR AUTUMN

As summer makes way for the dazzling colors of autumn, crops grow ripe for harvest and the wind begins to whisper of the coming winter. Most of the deciduous trees have already begun to prepare for winter by recycling the precious chlorophyll that allows them to harness sunlight and turn it into food. As the temperature drops, they break down their chlorophyll and store it for the next season, revealing the treasure trove of vibrant red, orange, and yellow hidden beneath. They go on to recycle these pigments as well and, when this process is complete, they shed their leaves.

In autumn, our bodies also begin to shift gears. The harvest brings with it an abundance of carbohydrate-rich foods, and we start to put on an extra layer of fat in a normal physiological process that once helped our ancestors survive the leaner months of winter when food was scarce. Like the trees, our bodies are designed to adjust to the seasons—and to the cycles of our lives.

During this transitional time, the weather is less predictable and storms more frequent, putting stress on our respiratory systems and causing conditions like asthma to flare up. Our immune systems step up a gear as seasonal infections begin to make their rounds, and children bring colds and viruses home from school. The shorter days begin to impact our moods, and those who are particularly sensitive may find this time of year difficult.[1]

Plant spirit allies for this season can help ease this transition and provide the courage we need to face the dark time ahead. Just as deciduous trees recycle the pigments in their leaves, we can use this time to gather our energy and convert the exuberance of summer into the wisdom that will see us through the darkness of winter.

Chapter 14

Mullein

Common names: *mullein, hag taper, Aaron's rod, candlewick*
Latin name: *Verbascum thapsus*
Family: *Scrophulariaceae*
Parts used: *leaves in spring, flowers in summer, roots after flowering*

Mullein stands straight and proud. It is taller than most herbs, with fuzzy lemon-yellow flowers that sprout all around the top. If you've ever spotted mullein growing in the wild, you know that it draws attention. Its magnificent spike can tower over even the tallest of plants. It's easy to see how this stately herb captured the folk imagination, showing up in myths and legends, and gaining a myriad of common names.

On a recent holiday in southern Spain, while walking along a beach path with my husband, I was greeted by a sea of flowering mullein. It filled me with joy to see it flourishing at a time of year when my flowers in Scotland were still far from blooming. Whenever I come upon an herbal ally in the wild, I am overwhelmed with gladness and delight, and I danced at the sight of this dear friend.

I made an impromptu offering of my hair to the Spirit of Mullein, thanking it for showing up for me, and picked three flowers to take home and dry for my altar. I had been feeling a bit overwhelmed, but having this unexpected meeting with a dear herbal ally made me feel grounded and set me back on my path.

Mullein has strong traditional associations with fire, and is also known as candlewick because its leaves were often used as lamp wicks before the introduction of cotton.[1] It is also known as hag's torch, because its tall spikes were dipped in tallow and used as torches by the Romans at funeral processions and other ceremonies to provide light and protection. These tall, fibrous stalks make ideal torches because they burn slowly and steadily. It is said that Ulysses himself was given a mullein torch to protect himself against the enchantments of the sorceress Circe. The ancient Celts believed that mullein could bring back children who were "away with the fairies," and they consumed it daily along with other herbs to improve longevity.[2]

Mullein taught me patience. Many of the herbs I work with are annuals. They grow in a single season, so I can harvest their medicine every year. But mullein is biennial and flowers in its second year. I have to wait a whole season before I can gather its delightful flowers, which have become a staple in my first aid cabinet. The flowers are slow to bloom and don't open all at once, so I must harvest them over several days rather than in one session.

Habitat

Mullein grows in well-drained, sandy, gravelly soils and is often found in disturbed areas like meadows, roadsides, and vacant lots. It prefers full sunlight, but can tolerate partial shade. The plant is adaptable and resilient, and thrives in diverse conditions. In the wild, mullein supports ecological restoration by colonizing open spaces and helping restore disturbed habitats.

Identification

Mullein is a biennial herb that flowers in its second year. In its first year, it grows in a rosette that hugs the ground, then it puts forth a tall, flowering spike in its second year. It usually produces a single spike, but I've also found plants with more than one. The spike is covered with individual fuzzy green flower buds that eventually open up to reveal five-lobed yellow flowers 12–35 mm (½–1") wide. The leaves are hairy and felt-like, giving this plant a downy white appearance. They become increasingly smaller as you go higher up the stalk. Common look-alikes include lamb's ear, comfrey, and foxglove.

Harvesting, Drying, and Storing

Harvest mullein leaves in either the first or second year, before the flower spikes start to form. The plant needs its leaves in the first year in order to grow flowers in the second, so be careful not to strip a plant of all its leaves. Harvest a few from each plant so that they can recover and continue growing and flowering.

Aim to collect the leaves when they are dry to the touch. This can be tricky, as they like to hold on to water longer than other plants. You will have a better chance of harvesting dry leaves late in the afternoon.

Pick the flowers individually late in the season. This ensures that the plant won't be damaged and can continue flowering. Only a few flowers open on a stalk each day, so you need to visit the plant every day or every other day when it's in bloom.

To dry the leaves, cut them into lateral strips 4–5 cm (1½–2") wide and lay them out flat on trays. Mullein attracts moisture from the air, so an airing cupboard is the best place to dry them passively. You can also dry them actively in a dehydrator set at 43°C (110F°) for eleven to twelve hours.

If you choose to dry the flowers, place the individual blossoms flat on trays and dry them the same way you would the leaves. The flowers take less time to dry than the leaves, so check them regularly. I usually work with fresh mullein flowers and infuse them in oil.

To dry the roots, clean them and slice them lengthwise into pieces that are approximately the size of matchsticks. You can dry roots passively, or in a dehydrator set to 43°C (110°F) for eleven to twelve hours. Roots are dry when they snap cleanly with no excessive bending, which can indicate that there is water left in the root.

Contraindications

The small hairs on mullein leaves can irritate mucous membranes. When working with the leaves in infusions, be sure to strain them with a fine mesh strainer before drinking or applying any preparations topically. Avoid mullein seeds, as they contain rotenone, a natural pesticide and insecticide produced by the plant.

Four Sacred Medicines

Mullein has many uses as a physical treatment, but also has strong mental, emotional, and spiritual healing properties.

Physical Medicine

Mullein leaves and flowers have an affinity with the respiratory and digestive systems. The roots also have a long history of being used for pain relief, especially for acute pain with nerve involvement. Topically, the leaves or roots can be made into a poultice to help support bone healing.

- *Respiratory tract*: Mullein is one of my top go-to herbs for all types of coughs and upper respiratory infections. This cooling, soothing herb is specific for dry, hard coughs when mucus is tacky and stuck, but I have also used it to treat coughs that are more productive. I use the flower-infused oil to treat ear infections, sore or itchy eyes and ears, and swollen glands that are the result of chronic illness or acute infection. It is especially good to have on hand in the winter to treat the increased incidence of respiratory issues associated with this season, which is estimated to be as high as 14 percent.[3]

- *Chronic coughs and asthma*: Mullein is mildly sedative, which accounts for its effectiveness in treating chronic or spasmodic coughs. The dried leaves were traditionally smoked to help ease asthma and lung congestion.

- *Digestive system*: Mullein's astringent action makes it effective for treating digestive tract bleeding, and acute and chronic diarrhea.

- *Nervous system*: Mullein root decoctions and tinctures have an affinity with the nervous system and are effective for easing back pain. As a nerve-pain remedy, mullein root combines well with St. John's Wort (*Hypericum perforatum*) and Jamaican dogwood (*Piscidia erythrina*) for ailments like Bell's palsy and trigeminal neuralgia. It can be used both topically and internally.

- *Urinary tract*: Mullein also has an affinity with the urinary tract and is useful for treating stress incontinence, when sneezing, coughing, bouncing, and running result in leaking urine.

Mental Medicine

If you are easily distracted and prone to "shiny object syndrome," mullein, with its upright stalk, can help you stay focused. With its mild sedative action, it is also very helpful for type-A personalities who find it difficult to relax and let go.

Emotional Medicine

Mullein can support you through intense emotional experiences and help you stay grounded and present to what is. It both softens hardness and hardens softness. It provides structure where there is a lack of boundaries, and soothes sharp edges where boundaries have turned into walls.

Spiritual Medicine

Mullein's association with fire and with Ulysses shows that this upright herbal ally will illuminate your path forward. If you are unsure or scared of taking the next step, it lights the way and provides a sense of safety and grounding. Burning mullein and decorating the entrances to homes with it invokes protection against unwanted energies. You can also call on its protective properties by carrying it on your person in a sachet or medicine pouch.

Working with Mullein

These three practices illustrate the many ways in which you can call upon this plant ally to heal, to protect, and to clarify intentions.

Practice: Mullein Flower Infused Oil

Mullein flower oil is often used for earaches and as a soothing skin remedy for general redness, pain, or inflammation. It is also effective for treating painful swollen glands. This particular method of infusing oil is straightforward and quick.

To make this oil, you will need:

- Fresh mullein flowers—enough to fill your chosen jar or container

- High-quality carrier oil, like olive oil, almond oil, or jojoba oil

- A double boiler or a heat-resistant bowl placed over a saucepan

- A clean, dry jar or container with a lid

- A fine mesh strainer or cheesecloth

- A dark glass bottle for storage (optional)

- A funnel (optional)

- A coffee filter (optional)

To avoid excess moisture in the flowers, pick them on a dry, sunny day. Be sure to shake or brush them off gently to remove any insects or debris. Allow the flowers to wilt for a few hours to reduce moisture content. This helps prevent mold during the infusion process.

Fill the bottom of a double boiler with water. If you don't have a double boiler, put a little water in a saucepan and place a heat-resistant bowl over it. Heat the water until it simmers gently, then place the wilted mullein flowers into the top of the double boiler or the heat-resistant bowl. Pour enough carrier oil over the flowers to cover them completely. Let the mixture simmer for three to four hours, making sure that the water in the bottom of the double boiler or pan does not evaporate completely. Stir occasionally to ensure an even infusion.

When the oil is sufficiently heated, remove the double boiler or pan from the heat and allow the mixture to cool slightly. Using a fine mesh strainer or cheesecloth, strain the oil into a clean, dry jar or container. Squeeze out as much oil as possible from the flowers. This part is messy, so I recommend wearing something with short sleeves. You can use the oil left on your hands to moisturize your arms!

Let the oil sit undisturbed for a few days so that any remaining sediment settles to the bottom. If you notice sediment building up in the bottom of the bottle, carefully pour the clear oil into another clean glass bottle using a funnel and leave the sediment behind. Cap the bottle tightly and label it with the date and contents. Stored in a cool, dark place, the oil should last for about a year.

To treat earaches, warm a few drops of the oil and test it on your skin first to make sure it's not too hot. Then apply gently into the ear canal using a dropper. If there is infection present, you can add several chopped, fresh garlic cloves to the oil for the last hour or two of infusion. For skin issues, apply the oil directly to the affected area to benefit from its soothing, pain-relieving, and anti-inflammatory properties.

Practice: Mullein Torches

Mullein torches, also known as witch tapers or hag tapers, have been used in rituals and ceremonies since ancient times.

To make these torches, you will need:

- Dried mullein stalks

- Approximately 450g (15 oz.) beeswax per stalk (this can be new or repurposed from old candles)

- A double boiler or a heat-resistant bowl and saucepan

- Grease-resistant paper

- Tongs or heat-resistant gloves

Collect mullein stalks at the end of summer once the flowers have dropped and the seeds are dispersing. Hang them to dry in a well-ventilated area for two to four weeks, until they are very dry.

Melt the beeswax in a double boiler or place a heat-resistant bowl over a pan with a little water in it. If you're repurposing old candles, make sure to remove any remnants like wicks. Cover your workspace with grease-resistant paper to catch any wax drips.

Pour the melted wax over the mullein stalks, making sure they are fully coated. Allow each layer of wax to dry before applying the next. Aim for about five layers to achieve a thick, even coating. If the wax starts to cool and solidify, reheat it as necessary. You can reuse any solidified wax drips from the earlier layers you poured.

Once the final layer of wax has dried, the torches are ready for use. To light, pinch off a small amount of wax from the tip to expose the dried mullein beneath and hold a flame to it until it ignites. Use the torches outdoors, away from flammable materials, children, and pets. It's best to place them in a pot filled with sand or soil, or stake them into the ground, as the wax will drip.

Always handle lit torches with care to prevent burns from both the flame and from dripping wax. Never leave burning torches unattended, and make sure they are completely extinguished when you are finished with them.

Practice: Ceremony to Clarify Your Path

Mullein torches are known for their protective and illuminating properties. In this ceremony, you use one to bring clarity and insight to your future path. These torches burn slowly and steadily, so you can work with the same torch for several ceremonies if necessary.

To perform this ceremony, you will need:

- A mullein torch (see page 216)

- Matches or a lighter

- A small pot filled with sand or soil in which to place the torch

- Your journal and a pen

Choose a quiet, comfortable outdoor location where you will not be disturbed. Set up an altar, arranging any seasonal flowers and herbs around it. Place the small pot filled with sand or soil in the center of your altar to hold the torch securely. Open your space in your usual way, calling upon the Spirit of Mullein.

Hold the mullein torch over the pot of sand or soil and light it, focusing on the flame and its illuminating energy. As the torch burns, recite an invocation to seek clarity on your path. You can use something like this or something you create yourself:

Spirit of Mullein,

Illuminate my path with the light of truth,

And grant me clarity and insight

So that I may know the way forward

That is for my best and highest good at this time.

Sit comfortably in front of the torch and gaze into the flame. Allow your mind to clear and focus on the question: "What is next on my path?" Spend some time in quiet meditation, observing any thoughts, images, or feelings that arise. If your mind wanders, simply give thanks to these thoughts and refocus on the flame.

When you feel complete, record any insights, messages, or feelings that came to you during the meditation in your journal. Reflect on what these impressions may mean for your future path. Write freely and let your thoughts flow. The goal is not perfect prose, so feel free to scribble as quickly as you can manage.

When you are ready, extinguish the torch safely by pushing the burning end into the sand or soil, making sure it is fully extinguished. Thank the Spirit of Mullein for its presence and guidance. Finally, state that your space is now closed.

Over the following days, spend some time integrating the insights you received. Consider any actions you can take based on the clarity you gained. Remember that action is the important final step of any ceremony!

Chapter 15

Elder

Common names: *elder, elderberry, elderflower*

Latin name: *Sambucus nigra*

Family: *Caprifoliaceae*

Parts used: *flowers in summer, berries in autumn*

Elder was one of those herbal allies that made me wait and work before I could connect with its medicine. Early in my plant spirit journey, I approached an elder tree on the property where I lived at the time. I carried out my usual rituals—I said "hello"; I introduced myself; I gave an offering. Then I asked for permission to work with its medicine. I'm not going to lie—I fully expected a resounding "yes." But I was summarily dismissed with a resounding "no."

At that point on my path, I didn't yet understand that I could inquire further, asking if there was something I needed to do to make myself ready. So I left feeling a little hurt and dejected. It took me a whole year to work up the courage to try again. This time, I knew that I could politely inquire as to my options if the answer was "no." I came prepared with some homemade rye bread as an offering and some butterflies in my stomach, hoping the answer would be positive.

But again, elder said "no." I took some breaths and leaned into the discomfort of once again having my request denied. Then I asked if the Spirit of Elder would ever allow me to work with it. This time, the answer was clear: "You are not ready yet; come back next year."

This wasn't quite enough to satisfy my curiosity, however, so I asked the plant spirit to be more specific. What steps did I need to take to make myself ready? "Connect with your heart space and learn from your intuition," the spirit replied.

Reflecting on these words, I saw that, although I was beginning to connect and learn directly from plants, I was still placing too much emphasis on books and information. My knowledge had not yet turned into wisdom, and I was not yet living a fully embodied and intuitive life. I was still using the accumulation of physical facts as a means to escape experiencing the fullness of life.

Fast-forward a number of years, and elder is now one of my key plant spirit allies. It doesn't hesitate to let me know when I am straying from my path and falling back into old habits. In plant spirit journeys, elder appears for me as a wizened old woman, one with a sharp tongue and a massive heart. She is not afraid to let me know when I'm out of line, but is also the first to provide protection and reassurance when I need it.

In Scotland, elder is seen as second only to rowan for its protective qualities against witchcraft, evil spells, and general negative energy. It was often planted at the back of a house, while rowan was planted at the front. It was understood that you had to be granted permission from the plant before gathering any part of it. Forget to do this, and dire consequences could ensue.

Hollow elder stems were once used as an instrument similar to panpipes. In fact, elder's first Latin name, *Sambucus*, comes from the Latin term for a musical instrument called a *sambuca*.

Habitat

Elder can be found in North and South America, Europe, and Asia, as well as in parts of the South Pacific. It is an opportunistic plant that grows in woods, hedges, scrub, wasteland, and cultivated ground. In Britain, it is often used for hedgerows because it grows quickly and can be trained to a desired shape.

Identification

Elder is a deciduous shrub or small tree that grows up to 6 m (20') tall and 6 m (20') wide. The bark of this tree is a light brown-gray, with a yellow color visible through cracks in the bark.

The light green and slightly serrated leaves are spear-shaped, 5–10 cm (½–2") long, and 3–5 cm (1–2") wide. They grow in opposing pairs, arranged in a feathery pattern of five to seven pairs along the stem. The flowers, which grow to 5–6 mm (¼") in diameter, each have five petals and appear in large, flat umbels that are 10–25 cm (4–10") in diameter.

The fruit, like the flowers, grows in large umbels. The glossy dark purple berries are small and almost perfectly round, measuring 5–6 mm (¼") in diameter. Elder fruit droops downward when ripe like a miniature bunch of grapes.

Harvesting, Drying, and Storing

Raw elderberries and flowers contain a poisonous cyanogenic glycoside called sambunigrin. This is found in the highest concentrations in the leaves and bark, and in lower concentrations in the berries, although I still don't recommended consuming the raw berries or juice. Cooking or drying causes the sambunigrin to break down and become harmless to the human body.

Harvest the whole umbel of flowers. Using secateurs, snip the head and place it facing down in your basket to allow any insects to escape. Don't wash elderflowers, as they will turn to mush and you will lose some of the medicinal pollen. You can wash the berries if you like.

To process the berries, place them in a bowl of fresh cold water and remove them from the stalks with your fingers or a fork. This is a labor-intensive but important part of the process, as the stalk can cause diarrhea if consumed. Be careful that as little of the stalk as possible finds its way into your final product. Once removed from the stalk, place the berries in another bowl of cold, fresh water and remove and discard any floating, unripe berries. The remaining berries are ready to dry or to process into a syrup or fresh tincture.

Dry flower umbels whole, and remove flowers from the stalk after you have dried them. Aim for dry, papery, crisp, still creamy-colored and intact blossoms. You can dry elderflowers passively, or using a dehydrator set to 42°C (107°F) for twelve hours or overnight.

ELDER

Contraindications

The bark and leaf of elder are strongly purgative and are no longer used internally. Because of the presence of cyanogenic glycosides, elder must not be consumed fresh. Once dried or processed into tinctures or syrups, however, the flowers and berries are a safe and well-tolerated herbal medicine.

Four Sacred Medicines

Elder has many medicinal uses and is especially effective in supporting you as you connect to your inner wisdom.

Physical Medicine

The physical medicine of elder is very healing and fortifying. Both the dried berries and flowers can be used internally, with the flowers being more effective at managing fevers and the berries having higher antiviral and immune-supporting properties.

- *Respiratory system*: Both berries and flowers can be used to ease the mucus and congestion associated with colds and rhinitis. If catarrhal deafness or a stubborn sinus infection is present, you can combine elder with plantain (*Plantago major/minor*) and eyebright (*Euphrasia officinalis*) in equal parts.

- *Fevers:* For fevers associated with coughs and colds, elder combines well in equal parts with peppermint and yarrow. You can sweeten the mixture with honey to improve the taste for children. Hot infusions of elderberry and elderflower are best for managing fever, while a cold flower infusion makes a lovely soothing eye wash for any type of irritation.

- *Coughs:* For dry, tight coughs (think whooping cough and bronchitis), combine elder in equal parts with red clover. For congested, mucus-filled coughs, combine it with goldenrod (*Solidago virgaurea*) and echinacea root (*Echinacea purpurea/angustifolia*).

- *Hayfever:* Elderflower pollen is very useful for managing hayfever. Carefully combine dried elderflowers with the pollen preserved in equal parts with nettle leaf (*Urtica dioica*) and plantain (*Plantago major/minor*) and start drinking it before the onset of allergy season.

ELDER

- *Inflammation*: Elderberries and elderflower both contain substances that work directly to reduce free radicals, leading to lower levels of inflammation and less cell damage. Elder is also directly anti-inflammatory, and the berries and flowers have long been used for joint pain and inflammation. You can use internal preparations like teas or tinctures, or external preparations like ointments. Another option is to bathe in water that contains elderberry extract.

Mental Medicine

Thanks to its expansive nature, elder can help you see a thorny situation from different perspectives and encourages you to step outside your ordinary worldview. It can also help you think through ancestral issues and family patterns, so you can make better choices for your own life.

Emotional Medicine

The outward and diffusive nature of elder helps you open up after you've been closed down. This supportive herb encourages you to rest and reconnect after difficult experiences have left you fearful and operating from a place of activation.

Spiritual Medicine

Elder spirit medicine is very powerful, but it is also very gentle. This plant spirit encourages you to turn inward, to see yourself clearly, and to connect with your inner wisdom. It often shows up in plant spirit journeys to give you the strength to follow your truth. It can clear blockages that cloud your intuition and inner knowing, and bring insight into the meaning of your dreams.

Working with Elder

Below you'll find a recipe and a ceremony that can put you in touch with this plant spirit and help you summon up its powerful medicine.

Practice: Elderberry Rob

This is an old-fashioned syrup that tastes delightful. It makes a lovely autumn and winter tonic when taken daily.

To make this syrup, you will need:

- 250ml (1 cup) dried elderberries

- 1 liter (4 cups) water

- 250ml (1 cup) honey

ELDER

- 1 cinnamon stick

- 4 cloves

- 2 cardamom pods

- 1 lemon, sliced

- 2½ cm (1") piece of fresh ginger, sliced

- A saucepan

- A fine mesh sieve or cheesecloth

- A sterilized bottle for storing

Rinse dried elderberries under cold water. In a saucepan, combine the berries, water, cinnamon, cloves, cardamom pods (split open to reveal the seeds), and ginger.

Bring the mixture to a gentle boil over medium-high heat, then reduce the heat to low and let the mixture simmer uncovered for about thirty minutes, stirring occasionally. After thirty minutes, remove the mixture from the heat and let it cool slightly, then strain it through a fine mesh sieve or cheesecloth into a clean container. Press down on the berries to extract as much liquid as possible.

Discard the solids and return the liquid to the saucepan. Stir in the honey until it's completely dissolved. Add the sliced lemon and place the saucepan back over a low heat. Warm the mixture gently for another five to ten minutes, stirring occasionally. Do not let it boil. Once warmed through, remove it from the heat and let it cool completely.

Transfer the mixture to a sterilized bottle or jar with a tight-fitting lid. You can add different spices to suit your taste. When winter starts to get you down, take one teaspoon daily, either off the spoon or mixed in warm water. You can also take up to three teaspoons daily at the onset of a cough or cold. This recipe will last up to three months if kept in the refrigerator.

Practice: Elder Ceremony for Expansion

Elder can help you expand your mind and see things from a new perspective. In this ceremony, I invite you to call on the mental medicine of elder to reimagine a long-standing problem in your life. To perform it, all you need is an umbel of elder flowers, or a photo or drawing if none are available. Find a quiet and comfortable space to sit or lie down, and be sure to bring your journal and a pen to record your experience.

Prepare yourself to enter a sacred space in your usual way. Open your space by calling on the Spirit of Elder to guide you. Sit comfortably and take several deep breaths to center yourself.

When you are ready, visualize the problem on which you'd like an expanded perspective. Really try to "see" this problem in your mind's eye. If you find it hard to visualize, you can sketch or draw it. Once you have the problem clearly in your mind, open your eyes and pick up the umbel of elderflowers. Notice how wide and spreading it is, with every white flower perfectly exposed to the light. Allow yourself to feel this expansive energy flowing into your mind and body.

Continue to gaze at the umbel, connecting to the Spirit of Elder. Notice if any new insights pop into your head related to the problem at hand. Can you "see" the problem differently when you connect to elder medicine?

When you feel complete, close your space in your usual way, giving thanks to the Spirit of Elder. Record your insights in your journal.

Chapter 16

Rose

Common name: *rose*
Latin name: *Rosa spp.*
Family: *Rosaceae*
Parts used: *flowers in summer, rosehips in autumn*

Rarely has a flower captured the human imagination the way the rose has. It has been seen as a muse, a symbol, and a metaphor. It has been a mainstay of art, poetry, and design. The Scottish poet Robert (or Rabbie, as we call him in Scotland) Burns wrote about roses in over sixty poems and songs. Rose has been hailed as a savior of nations in times of hardship, and supports a giant industry that produces over one billion stems a year.[1] I'm not sure if any other plant comes close to having the breadth and depth of influence that the rose has had.

My personal relationship with roses goes back to early childhood, when their scent fascinated me. I spent hours sniffing the roses my dad grew in our gardens. My siblings and I made rose perfume in his old weeding bucket and sold it to my mum, and to any other unsuspecting adult who lingered long enough to talk to us.

Roses are often thought of as delicate flowers, portrayed in poetry as perfumed and trembling under a lover's gaze. Yet roses are bold and strong. Their thorns cut deep, providing protection for the precious seeds held in the rosehips. The roots hold fast, and the final casings for the seeds are full of irritating hairs that teach ultimate patience when deseeding. The flowers bloom fully and unapologetically for all to see.

After my father died, we transplanted two of his favorite rose bushes into the garden behind the house where my mum now lives. It was a monumental task, and one that I vastly underestimated. In the attempt to remove the shrubs, I broke two of my mother's garden forks and fell on my back, covering myself in soil and scratches. It took me most of the day to dig the bushes out. In the process, I learned that you can find laughter amid grief, and joy where there is pain. This is one of the key lessons of rose. I was living the medicine in real time, being shown it in a way that I would never forget.

I continue to be transfixed by roses. To this day, if I see a rose, whether in a stately garden or growing wild, I feel compelled to stop and breathe in its fragrance. If it's been raining, I collect the raindrops off the flowers and use them as a refreshing facial treatment. Rose is now a key plant spirit ally for me. I find its medicine particularly helpful when I am dealing with boundary issues, or if I am involved in an argument where the original intent is lost, and trauma and conditioned responses have taken the reins.

Habitat

Roses are native to the temperate regions of the Northern Hemisphere. China and what was once known as the Fertile Crescent—which includes present-day Iraq, Syria, Lebanon, Israel, Palestine, Jordan, parts of Egypt, Turkey, and Iran— have been breeding roses for thousands of years. They thrive in sunny, well-drained soil and particularly like clay soils. Wild roses (*Rosa canina*) and Japanese roses (*Rosa rugosa*) grow in hedgerows in the UK.

Identification

Today, there are hundreds of rose species and thousands of cultivars. They come in various forms, including more traditional shrubs, climbers, and miniature pot plants. Their stems are usually spiked with sharp thorns. Their glossy green leaves have toothed edges.

Rose flowers vary in size and shape. Their colors range from pastel pink to peach and cream, as well as vibrant yellow, orange, and red. The shapes of rose flowers vary widely, from the simple, flat dog rose to intricate rosette formations. All roses can be used medicinally providing they have not been sprayed with pesticides.

Rosehips—the rose plant's fruit—develop from the pollinated flowers. They are round or oval, varying in size and color depending on the rose. They possess a smooth, glossy exterior and contain numerous tiny, hairy seeds encased in a fleshy pulp.

Harvesting, Drying, and Storing

When rose blossoms have just opened or are in the process of opening, cut the whole flower off beneath the stem at the green calyx. Handle them gently so you don't bruise and discolor the petals. This is best done on a sunny day so that the blossoms are not saturated with moisture, as this will increase the time they need to dry.

Don't wash the flowers, as they will turn to mush. You can wash the rosehips, however, by placing them in a bowl of fresh, cold water. Remove any that are significantly discolored and discard. Using a small, sharp knife, cut the top and tail off the hip, then split it in half and scrape out the seeds and little hairs. This is an important step, as the hairs are irritating if ingested. I recommend doing this wearing cotton gloves, as the hairs will make you itch!

If you are drying rosehips to prepare a tincture or syrup, you can skip the step of cutting open and scraping out seeds and hairs. But be sure to strain the tincture or syrup through muslin or cheesecloth before using it. For all other purposes, I recommend removing the insides first. It takes time, but my experience has shown me that waiting to do this job until the rosehips are dry can be a massive pain. It is most definitely a labor of love.

To dry the flowers, remove them from the green calyx first. Gently tease the petals apart and dry them flat. Aim for dry, papery, crisp, but still vibrantly colored flowers. You can dry rose petals passively, or set a dehydrator to 42°C (107°F) and leave them for twelve hours or overnight.

ROSE

You can dry rosehips passively, or with a dehydrator set to 57–60°C (135–140°F). Depending on the size and moisture content of the rosehips, drying can take anywhere from six to twelve hours. Check them periodically to prevent overdrying. The rosehips should be hard and brittle, with no remaining moisture. They should snap easily when bent.

Contraindications

Avoid rose petals during pregnancy, but rosehips are safe to use.

Four Sacred Medicines

The Spirit of Rose has a long history in folklore and legend. In addition to its physical properties, it is known to bring solace to those in grief and to support relationships of all kinds.

Physical Medicine

The physical properties of the rose relate primarily to internal ailments like inflammation and problems with the digestive and reproductive systems.

- *Digestive system*: Rose can help reestablish a healthy microbiome (the helpful bacteria that live in your gut). It also supports the liver by increasing bile production and assisting in the metabolization of hormones and toxins.

- *Inflammation*: Rose flowers and hips both contain substances that help to reduce free radicals, leading to lower levels of inflammation and less cell damage. They are both directly anti-inflammatory. Rosehips have been proven to reduce the pain associated with osteoarthritis and rheumatoid arthritis. This anti-inflammatory action can also be helpful in cases of general inflammation, like irritable bowel syndrome and ulcers.

- *Menstrual health*: Rose can help lighten menstrual flow and decrease the pain associated with it. It can regulate heavy, painful, or irregular periods. It's particularly indicated where ovulation is unpredictable, because it helps to establish regular patterns and healthy flow. It eases headaches and constipation if they are present.

- *Nervous system*: Rose can restore a tense and burned-out nervous system, especially when insomnia, depression, irritability, and fatigue are present. It supports the mood changes associated with menopause and perimenopause.

Mental Medicine

If you feel easily irritated by others (or by yourself!), rose can help you uncover why, so you can take steps to feel more expansive and settled. It eases the bitterness and harsh thoughts that come with disappointment and encourages you to let love and compassion back into your mind.

Emotional Medicine

If you have closed your heart after being disappointed or abandoned, rose can help you open it again and connect you to a sense of safety and nurturance. Like hawthorn, rose can help you through the grieving process. It is especially effective in dealing with old, buried grief that you have processed mentally, but not emotionally or physically.

Spiritual Medicine

The spirit medicine of the rose is associated with love. Making a necklace from dried rosehips is said to attract love. The Spirit of Rose can lead you on a heart-opening journey to self-love and connection with the unconditional love of nature. If you are locked down and avoiding connection, but yearn for meaningful relationships, rose can gently open you up. Rose petal tea supports prophetic dreaming when taken before sleep, so you can receive communication from your spirit guides.

While the rose represents love and beauty, its thorns remind you to guard and protect your inner space. They symbolize the importance of setting boundaries to safeguard your heart and personal space. They teach you that it's okay to be open and loving, but it's wise to have mechanisms that protect you from harm and maintain your integrity.

Working with Rose

There are many ways to work with rose—both traditional and modern. Below are three examples of how to reach out to this powerful plant spirit.

Practice: Rosehip Electuary

Electuaries are one of my favorite old-fashioned ways to prepare and preserve herbs. Aside from their fascinating name, they also taste delicious—something that is not that common in herbal medicine!

Electuaries are finely powdered herbs mixed with honey. They can vary in consistency from a runny liquid to a thick paste, depending on how much herb you blend with the honey—and this comes down to individual preference. They are useful for anyone who cannot (or will not) tolerate strong flavors or bitter herbs.

To make this recipe, you will need:

- 85g (3 oz.) dried rosehips

- 300ml (1¼ cups) runny honey

- 500ml (1 pint) capacity sterilized canning jar

If your rosehips still contain seeds or hairs, cut them in half and deseed them first. I recommend wearing gloves for this.

This recipe requires runny honey. If your honey is solid, gently warm it to liquefy it, but avoid overheating. Grind or chop the rosehips into a rough powder and place them in a mixing bowl.

Pour the honey over the herbs and mix well to form a thick paste. Then store the paste in a sterilized jar.

That's all there is to it! Take by the spoonful daily as an excellent source of vitamins and minerals, or add to your herbal tea for a flavor boost. Store in a cool, dark place and use within six months.

Practice: Rosewater

Because floral water made from rose petals is topically anti-inflammatory and anti-microbial, it is very soothing for hot, itchy skin conditions.[2] You can work with it as part of your daily skincare routine, as it makes an effective skin toner.

The essential oils that give rose its distinctive aroma have an uplifting effect on mood, so this mixture can also be used as a spray in your home or on your pillow to promote relaxation and improve mood. I also use it in ceremonies to anoint myself or sacred objects.

This recipe will not work with roses that don't have a fragrance. And be sure to choose roses that are organic and pesticide-free.

To make this floral water, you will need:

- Fresh, scented rose petals

- A large pot with a lid (preferably transparent)

- A small heat-resistant bowl

- Ice cubes

- Spring water

Place the pot on the stove and put the small heat-resistant bowl in the center of it. Add rose petals around the side of the bowl, enough to create an even layer that comes approximately halfway up the side of the bowl.

Pour water over the petals until they are fully covered, making sure that the water level does not reach the top of the bowl. Place the pot lid upside down on the bowl and fill the inverted lid with ice cubes. Heat the pot gently on low to medium heat. As the water in the pot heats up, steam will rise and hit the cold lid, then condense and drip back into the bowl.

Continue heating until you collect enough floral water in the bowl (about thirty to forty-five minutes). Replenish the ice as needed. Allow the floral water to cool, then pour it into a sterilized bottle and store it in the refrigerator.

Homemade floral water will last approximately a week if refrigerated. To extend its life, add one teaspoon of vodka or other high-proof alcohol per cup. This will help prevent microbial growth and extend the storage life up to a month.

Practice: Ceremony—It's All About Boundaries

This ceremony is designed to help you establish, maintain, or soften personal boundaries by working with the Spirit of Rose. Personal boundaries are essential for maintaining healthy relationships and personal well-being. They define your limits and communicate to others what is acceptable behavior and what is not. Without clear and effective boundaries, feelings of resentment and burnout can build up.

To perform this ceremony, you will need:

- Rosewater (see page 243)

- Fresh rose petals

- A candle

- A small bowl

- Your journal and a pen

- Comfortable seating

- Soft background music (optional)

Gather your materials and choose a quiet, comfortable location where you won't be disturbed. Place the rosewater, fresh rose petals, and candle on your plant spirit altar. Open your sacred space in your usual way, and be sure to include the Spirit of Rose in your opening invocation.

Sit comfortably and take a few deep breaths to center yourself. Light the candle to signify the beginning of the ceremony, and reflect on your intention. Do you want to strengthen your boundaries? Soften them? Find a balance? Feel the presence of Mother Earth beneath you. You are supported and protected by all of nature.

Pour a small amount of rosewater into the bowl. Hold the bowl in your hands and set an intention for the rosewater to support your boundary work. Take a handful of fresh rose petals and, one by one, dip them in the rosewater and place them around you in a circle. As you place each petal, silently affirm your intention. For example: "My boundaries are firm when needed." Or "My boundaries are not walls; they are flexible and match my needs." Sit within the circle of rose petals and reflect on your intention. Write down any thoughts, feelings, or insights that arise in your journal.

Dip your fingers in the rosewater and gently anoint your forehead, your heart, and your wrists. As you anoint each area, affirm your commitment to honoring your boundaries. Close your eyes and take a few deep breaths. Visualize the protective mantle of rose helping you to hold your boundaries.

Thank the Spirit of Rose for its guidance and support. Take a moment to feel gratitude for the insights and assistance you received. Extinguish the candle, signifying the end of the ceremony. Collect the rose petals and, if possible, return them to nature by burying them or scattering them in a garden. Store the remaining rosewater in a cool, dark place for future use.

Conclusion

Plant Spirit Allies for Life

As you move through the cycle of seasons, new plant spirit allies will begin to make themselves known to you in ways you may not have noticed before you embarked on this path. A flower may catch your eye on the side of a trail. You may find dried seed pods on the ground that lead you to a new herbal friend. An unfamiliar tree may beckon, its branches whispering in the wind. Pale green shoots in your garden may invite you to look closer.

Each new encounter with an herb is an opportunity for curiosity and wonder, and these experiences only deepen the longer you work with plant spirit herbalism. Far from thinking you "know" plants, you realize that there are always more layers to discover. Although you may start out by resonating with one aspect of a plant's medicine, over time you may find yourself drawn to a different one. Its physical medicine may lead you to its emotional properties. Its mental associations may connect you to its spiritual powers. Ultimately, you find yourself in a holistic relationship that encompasses all aspects of your being.

Our plant allies can give us encouragement in times of doubt, joy in times of sorrow, and comfort in times of uncertainty. Just as plants grow—pushing their roots down into the earth and unfurling their leaves to drink in the sunlight they need to thrive—they likewise support our growth as human beings as we reach down and rise up. Through ceremony, ritual, and plain old paying attention, we can invite their healing energy to flow into our lives. Meanwhile, we participate in our own healing through the care and respect we show to our plant friends.

May you go forth and find plant allies to guide, support, and inspire you through all the seasons of your life. And may you never be too busy to kick off your shoes, walk into the garden, and be delighted by what you find.

Acknowledgments

This book would not have been possible without the brave, trailblazing herbalists who have gone before me. There are too many to name, but many have risked their livelihoods and lives by practicing herbalism.

To my husband, Josh: thank you for your love, humor, and patience and for keeping the home fires burning when I was deep in writing land and not fit for much else.

To my beautiful children Hamish and Aonghus: you push me to be a better person and have helped me rediscover my sense of adventure. Your love has forever changed me.

To Rhonda: thank you for your bravery in breaking down barriers and for your encouragement when I doubted myself.

To Mum and Dad: despite many hardships and tough times, you kept going and kept trying. Thank you for raising me with the eyes to appreciate the beauty in unexpected places and teaching me to never accept substandard coffee.

To Jayne: you showed up even when you were already juggling many things, providing care and nurturing for the boys so I could meet my deadlines.

To Leo: your steady, no-nonsense advice has made me a better writer and herbalist.

To all those at Hierophant Publishing who have contributed to making this book what it is: thank you for taking a chance and for your candor, flexibility, and patience with a new author.

To the plants, my mentors and guiding lights: thank you for trusting me with your stories.

Appendix

Opening and Closing Sacred Space

Whether you are preparing to conduct a sensory tea ceremony or embark on a plant spirit journey, knowing how to open and close sacred space is an essential step. This is a basic guide for both.

Opening Sacred Space

Although setting sacred space can be as elaborate as you like, at its most basic it simply means invoking qualities of protection and benevolence before engaging in spiritual work. The care you put into setting sacred space before a journey or ritual is just as important as the journey or ritual itself, so take your time and don't rush it.

Below, I share basic instructions for opening sacred space. You can adapt these to suit your own needs and preferences, allowing your space-setting ritual to evolve over time.

Step 1: Gather Your Tools

First, gather any tools or materials you will need to complete the task, ritual, or journey you have in mind: for example, herbs, scissors, a rattle, a lighter, or a blanket. Take care in the way you handle each object, imbuing them with the spirit of love, respect, and protection. The care with which you gather and arrange your tools and materials will have a dramatic effect on your peace of mind during the ritual or journey to come.

Step 2: Set Your Intention

An intention is a simple statement of purpose for the action, ritual, or journey you are undertaking. For example, if you are making an herbal tincture, your intention may be something like, "May this tincture bring good health to all those who consume it." If you are undertaking a plant spirit journey, your intention may be something like, "May I meet the Spirit of Elder to gain insight into my relationship with my family."

When setting sacred space, you can speak your intention out loud, think it silently, or write it on a card. Commit to your intention and resist the temptation to change it halfway through; remember, you can always do another ritual or journey on a different intention.

254   APPENDIX

Step 3: Prepare Your Body and Mind

The next step in setting sacred space is to release any mental worries or physical tensions that may distract you from your spiritual work. This often means making a ritual gesture to signify that you are temporarily setting aside your day-to-day concerns: for example, burning some fragrant dried herbs, shaking a rattle, or taking a series of deep, cleansing breaths. Doing this will ensure that you can stay relaxed and focused for the duration of your ceremony, ritual, or journey.

Step 4: Make Your Space-Opening Invocation

An invocation is a form of sacred speech which can be used to call in the protection of a specific deity, or to summon qualities such as love, compassion, and wisdom. When practicing plant spirit herbalism, you may wish to invoke a specific herbal ally. You can also call on natural elements such as the wind and ocean, your ancestors, or any deities who inspire you. An invocation can be as poetic or straightforward as you like, and can range from long and elaborate to concise but heartfelt. The important thing is to speak from the heart, allowing the qualities you are invoking to manifest in your own body and spirit.

At the end of your invocation, make a statement such as "This space is clear, this space is open." You are now ready to conduct your ritual or embark on your plant spirit journey.

Closing Sacred Space

Closing sacred space allows you to transition smoothly from a ritual or journey back into your ordinary life. Although it may be tempting to remain in a dreamy, ceremonial state of mind all the time, this can eventually drain you and make it difficult to attend to your more mundane responsibilities. I teach all my students the importance of disconnecting, rather than keeping the portal open all the time.

When I am finished with a sensory tea ceremony, plant spirit journey, or other ritual, I always state, "This space is now closed." I then thank all the beings who were present for my experience, such as the plant allies I invoked during the space-setting ritual. Finally, I fold up my blanket, blow out my candle, and complete any other tasks or gestures that indicate the ceremony is complete.

Index of Practices

Part II: Plant Spirit Allies for Winter

Chapter 5: Calendula

Hot Calendula Flower Infusion   81

Healing Calendula Sitz Bath   81

Calendula Healing Ceremony   82

Chapter 6: Dandelion

Dandelion Root Tincture   92

Italian Dandelion Soup (Cicoria)   93

Dandelion Herbal Amulet   94

Chapter 7: Rosemary

Rosemary and Sage Infused Wine   107

Rosemary Smoke-Cleansing Ceremony   108

Part III: Plant Spirit Allies for Spring

Chapter 8: Nettle

Nettle Leaf Pesto   125

Spring Greens Vinegar   127

Nettle Ceremony for Cleansing and Renewal   129

Chapter 9: Cleavers

Spring Cleansing Infusion   137

Cleavers Coffee   138

Cleavers Talisman Ceremony   139

Chapter 10: Wild Oat

Baking Bannocks   151

Tasty Oatstraw Tea Blend   153

Oat Gratitude Ceremony   153

Part IV: Plant Spirit Allies for Summer

Chapter 11: Hawthorn

Hawberry Ketchup   167

Hawthorn Flower Essence   168

Hawthorn Ceremony—Be Here Now   171

Chapter 12: Yarrow

Yarrow First Aid Powder   185

Yarrow Medicine Pouch   185

Chapter 13: Lemon Balm

Aromatic Lemon Balm Syrup   197

Lemon Balm Bath Ritual   198

Part V: Plant Spirit Allies for Autumn

Chapter 14: Mullein

Mullein Flower Infused Oil   213

Mullein Torches   216

Ceremony to Clarify Your Path   217

Chapter 15: Elder

Elderberry Rob   229

Elder Ceremony for Expansion   231

Chapter 16: Rose

Rosehip Electuary   242

Rosewater   243

Ceremony—It's All About Boundaries   245

Recommended Reading

Hundreds of books have been written on herbalism and plant spirit medicine. The ones I list here were written by herbalists who have been an inspiration to me in my own work. They are all books that I own and use regularly. They are all books that I love and trust.

These resources are a mix of spirit and science, of wisdom and modern medical practice. They are ideal for beginners, as well as those who already work with herbs and are interested in exploring the spiritual and energetic aspects of plant healing. I am confident they will expand your understanding and connection with the art of herbal medicine.

Cowan, Eliot. *Plant Spirit Medicine: A Journey into the Healing Wisdom of Plants* (Sounds True, 2014). Takes readers on a journey into the healing wisdom of plants and the practice of plant spirit medicine.

Easley, Thomas, and Steven Horne. *The Modern Herbal Dispensatory: A Medicine Making Guide* (North Atlantic Books, 2016). Provides a comprehensive guide to making herbal medicines and offers insights into the modern herbal dispensary. Includes useful insights into herbal energetics.

Green, James. *The Herbal Medicine Makers Handbook: A Home Manual* (Crossing Press, 2000). Excellent resource for those wanting to take a deeper dive into making their own herbal medicines.

Guyett, Carole. *Sacred Plant Initiations: Communicating with Plants for Healing and Higher Consciousness* (Bear & Company, 2015). Delves into the practice of communicating with plants for healing and expanding consciousness.

Heckels, Fiona, and Karen Lawton. *The Sensory Herbal Handbook: Connect with the Medicinal Power of Your Local Plants* (Watkins Publishing, 2019). Focuses on connecting with easy-to-find plants and their medicinal and magical properties.

Hoffmann, David. *Holistic Herbal: A Safe and Practical Guide to Making and Using Herbal Medicine* (Thorsons, 1990). A practical guide for making and using herbal medicine in a safe and holistic manner.

—————. *The Herbal Handbook: A User's Guide to Medical Herbalism* (Inner Traditions, 1999). User-friendly guide that provides an introduction to medical herbalism and offers practical advice on using herbs for healing purposes.

Kimmerer, Robin Wall. *Braiding Sweetgrass: Indigenous Wisdom, Scientific Knowledge, and the Teachings of Plants* (Milkweed Editions, 2015). This series of essays combines scientific botany with Indigenous teachings to reframe how we view the natural world.

McIntyre, Anne. *The Complete Woman's Herbal: A Manual of Healing Herbs and Nutrition for Personal Well-being and Family Care* (Henry Holt, 1994). Focuses on herbal remedies and treatments specifically tailored for women's health and well-being.

Mills, Simon Y, and Kerry Bone. *The Dictionary of Modern Herbalism: A Comprehensive Guide to Practical Herbal Therapy* (Healing

Arts Press, 2003). Comprehensive guide that serves as a reference for practical herbal therapy.

Montgomery, Pam. *Plant Spirit Healing: A Guide to Working with Plant Consciousness* (Bear & Company, 2008). Provides guidance on working with the consciousness of plants for healing purposes.

Wood, Matthew. *The Book of Herbal Wisdom: Using Plants as Medicines* (North Atlantic Books, 1997). Explores the use of plants as medicines, connecting with shamanism for direct revelation of the medicine of herbs. Provides wisdom and insights from the author's experience as an herbalist.

Notes

Chapter 1: Rituals of Connection

1. Chowdhury, Sutanu Dutta, Subhasish Pramanik, Koena Bhattacharjee, and Lakshmi Kanta Mondal. "Effects of Lunar Cycle on Fasting Plasma Glucose, Heart Rate and Blood Pressure in Type 2 Diabetic Patients," *Chronobiology International* 38, no. 2 (December 2020): 270–277, https://doi.org/10.1080/07420528.2020.1842754.

2. Uddin, Mohy, Aldilas Achmad Nursetyo, Usman Iqbal, Phung-Anh Nguyen, Wen-Shan Jian, Yu-Chan Li, and Shabbir Syed-Abdul. "Assessment of Effects of Moon Phases on Hospital Outpatient Visits: An Observational National Study," *AIMS Public Health* 10, no. 2 (May 2023): 324-332, https://doi.org/10.3934/publichealth.2023024.

3. Cajochen, Christian, Songül Altanay-Ekici, Mirjam Münch, Sylvia Frey, Vera Knoblauch, and Anna Wirz-Justice. "Evidence that the Lunar Cycle Influences Human Sleep," *Current Biology* 23, no. 15 (August 2013): 1485-1488, https://doi.org/10.1016/j.cub.2013.06.029.

Chapter 5: Calendula

1. Grieve, Maud. *A Modern Herbal*. Dover Publications, 1971.

2. Givol, Or, Rachel Kornhaber, Denis Visentin, Michelle Cleary, Josef Haik, and Moti Harats. "A Systematic Review of *Calendula officinalis* Extract for Wound Healing," *Wound Repair and Regeneration* 27, no. 5 (September/October 2019): 548–561, https://doi.org/10.1111/wrr.12737.

3. Khairnar, Mayur Sudhakar, Babita Pawar, Pramod Pashram Marawar, and Ameet Mani. "Evaluation of *Calendula officinalis* as an Anti-Plaque and Anti-Gingivitis Agent," *Journal of Indian Society of Periodontology* 17, no. 6 (November–December 2013): 741–747, https://doi.org/10.4103/0972-124X.124491.

4. Ahmed, Sheikh Rashel, Muhammad Fazle Rabbee, Anindita Roy, Rocky Chowdhury, Anik Banik, Khadizatul Kubra, Mohammed Mehadi Hassan Chowdhury, and Kwang-Hyun Baek. "Therapeutic Promises of Medicinal Plants in Bangladesh and Their Bioactive Compounds Against Ulcers and Inflammatory Diseases," *Plants* 10, no. 7 (July 2021): 1348, https://doi.org/10.3390/plants10071348.

Chapter 7: Rosemary

1. Samman, Samir, Brittmarie Sandström, Maja Bjørndal Toft, Klaus Bukhave, Mikael Jensen, Sven S. Sørensen, and Marianne Hansen. "Green Tea or Rosemary Extract Added to Foods Reduces Nonheme-Iron Absorption," *American Journal of Clinical Nutrition* 73, no. 3 (March 2001): 607–612, https://doi.org/10.1093/ajcn/73.3.607.

2. Rašković, Aleksandar, Isidora Milanović, Nebojša Pavlović, Tatjana Ćebović, Saša Vukmirović, and Momir Mikov. "Antioxidant Activity of Rosemary (*Rosmarinus officinalis L..*) Essential Oil and Its Hepatoprotective Potential," *BMC Complementary and Alternative Medicine* 14 (July 2014): 225, https://doi.org/10.1186/1472-6882-14-225.

3. Bone, Kerry, and Simon Mills. *Principles and Practices of Phytotherapy* (2nd ed.). Churchill Livingstone Elsevier, 2013.

4. Bozin, Biljana, Neda Mimica-Dukic, Isidora Samojilik, and Emilija Jovin. "Antimicrobial and Antioxidant Properties of Rosemary and Sage (*Rosmaris officinalis L. and Salvia officinalis L., Lamiaceae*) Essential Oils," *Journal of Agricultural and Food Chemistry* 55, no. 19 (August 2007): 7879–7885, https://doi.org/10.1021/jf0715323.

5. Bone and Mills. *Principles and Practices of Phytotherapy.*

6. Diego, Miguel A., Nancy Aaron Jones, Tiffany Field, Maria Hernandez-rief, Saul Schanberg, Cynthia Kuhn, Mary Galamaga, Virginia McAdam, and Robert Galamaga. "Aromatherapy Positively Affects Mood, EEG Patterns of Alertness and Math Computations." *International Journal of Neuroscience* 96, no. 3–4 (July 1998): 217–224, https://doi.org/10.3109/00207459808986469.

Part III: Plant Spirit Allies for Spring
1. Wohlleben, Peter. *The Hidden Life of Trees.* Greystone Books, 2016.

Chapter 8: Nettle

1. Milliken, William, and Sam Bridgewater. *Flora Celtica: Plants and People in Scotland*. Birlinn Limited, 2004.

2. Vickery, Roy. *Vickery's Folk Flora: An A–Z of the Folklore and Uses of British and Irish Plants*. Weidenfeld & Nicolson, 2019.

Chapter 10: Wild Oat

1. Paudel, Devendra, Bandana Dhungana, Melanie Caffe, and Padmanaban Krishnan. "A Review of Health-Beneficial Properties of Oats," *Foods* 10, no. 11 (October 2021): 2591, https://doi.org/10.3390/foods10112591.

Chapter 11: Hawthorn

1. Vickery, Roy. *Vickery's Folk Flora: An A–Z of the Folklore and Uses of British and Irish Plants*. Weidenfeld & Nicolson, 2019.

Chapter 12: Yarrow

1. Carmichael, Alexander, ed. *Carmina Gadelica (Charms of the Gaels): Hymns and Incantations*. Floris Books, 1994.

Part V: Plant Spirit Allies for Autumn

1. Xu, Lyuan, Soyoung Choi, Yu Zhao, Muwei Li, Baxter P. Rogers, Adam Anderson, John C. Gore, Yurui Ga, and Zhaohua Ding. "Seasonal Variations of Functional Connectivity of Human Brains," *Scientific Reports* 13 (October 2023): 16898, https://doi.org/10.1038/s41598-023-43152-4.

Chapter 14: Mullein

1. Grieve, Maud. *A Modern Herbal*. Dover Publications, 1971.

2. MacLeod, Sharon Paice. *Celtic Myth and Religion*. McFarland & Company, 2011.

3. Dales, R. E., I. Schweitzer, J. H. Toogood, M. Drouin, W. Yang, J. Dolovich, and J. Boulet. "Respiratory Infections and the Autumn Increase in Asthma Morbidity," *European Respiratory Journal* 9, no. 1 (January 1996): 72–77, https://doi.org/10.1183/09031936.96.09010072.

Chapter 16: Rose

1. "Year of the Rose." National Garden Bureau. Accessed July 20, 2024, https://ngb.org/year-of-the-rose/.

2. Maruyama, Naho, Shigeru Tansho-Nagakawa, Chizuru Miyazaki, Kazuyuki Shimomura, Yasuo Ono, and Shigeru Abe. "Inhibition of Neutrophil Adhesion and Antimicrobial Activity by Diluted Hydrosol Prepared from *Rosa damascena*," *Biological and Pharmacological Bulletin* 40, no. 2 (2017): 161–168, https://doi.org/10.1248/bpb.b16-00644. Erratum in *Biological and Pharmacological Bulletin* 40, no. 4 (2017): 546, https://doi.org/10.1248/bpb.b17-e4004.

About the Author

Wendy Dooner has immersed herself in the world of plants and herbalism for over two decades. She holds a bachelor's degree in herbal medicine from Napier University, and has completed extensive postgraduate professional training, including a three-year course in advanced shamanic practice. She lives in Kirriemuir, Scotland. Visit her at www.wendydooner.com.

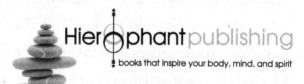

San Antonio, TX
www.hierophantpublishing.com